Technical Fundamentals of Radiology and CT

Technical Fundamentals of Radiology and CT

Guillermo Avendaño Cervantes
University of Valparaiso, Chile

IOP Publishing, Bristol, UK

© IOP Publishing Ltd 2016

All rights reserved. No part of this publication may be reproduced, stored in a retrieval system or transmitted in any form or by any means, electronic, mechanical, photocopying, recording or otherwise, without the prior permission of the publisher, or as expressly permitted by law or under terms agreed with the appropriate rights organization. Multiple copying is permitted in accordance with the terms of licences issued by the Copyright Licensing Agency, the Copyright Clearance Centre and other reproduction rights organisations.

Permission to make use of IOP Publishing content other than as set out above may be sought at permissions@iop.org.

Guillermo Avendaño Cervantes has asserted his right to be identified as the author of this work in accordance with sections 77 and 78 of the Copyright, Designs and Patents Act 1988.

ISBN   978-0-7503-1212-7 (ebook)
ISBN   978-0-7503-1213-4 (print)
ISBN   978-0-7503-1214-1 (mobi)

DOI   10.1088/978-0-7503-1212-7

Version: 20160501

IOP Expanding Physics
ISSN 2053-2563 (online)
ISSN 2054-7315 (print)

British Library Cataloguing-in-Publication Data: A catalogue record for this book is available from the British Library.

Published by IOP Publishing, wholly owned by The Institute of Physics, London

IOP Publishing, Temple Circus, Temple Way, Bristol, BS1 6HG, UK

US Office: IOP Publishing, Inc., 190 North Independence Mall West, Suite 601, Philadelphia, PA 19106, USA

Dedicated to biomedical engineering students, for choosing a specialty with the highest social utility

Contents

Preface	**xvi**
Acknowledgement	**xvii**
Author biography	**xviii**

1	**The basics of x-rays**	**1-1**
1.1	What are x-rays?	1-1
1.2	Characteristics and properties of x-rays	1-2
1.3	Substances and x-rays	1-3
1.4	The effect of x-rays on radiographic film	1-4
	References	1-5
2	**Radiographic quality**	**2-1**
2.1	Properties of radiographic quality	2-1
	2.1.1 Density	2-1
	2.1.2 Contrast	2-1
	2.1.3 Definition	2-1
	2.1.4 Distortion	2-2
2.2	Quality control factors	2-2
2.3	Density and current	2-3
2.4	The relationship between current and time	2-3
2.5	Other factors affecting density	2-4
	2.5.1 Focus–film distance	2-4
	2.5.2 Films and intensifying screens	2-5
	2.5.3 Anti-scatter grids	2-5
2.6	Kilovolts and contrast	2-6
2.7	Other factors controlling the contrast	2-7
	2.7.1 Grids	2-7
	2.7.2 Collimation and restrictions	2-7
	2.7.3 Filtering	2-7
	2.7.4 Film	2-7
	2.7.5 Film processing	2-7
	2.7.6 Screens	2-7
	2.7.7 The patient	2-7

2.8	Definition	2-8
	2.8.1 Deformation by movement	2-8
	2.8.2 Geometric deformation	2-8
	2.8.3 Focus–film distance	2-9
	2.8.4 The irradiated material	2-9
	2.8.5 Quantum traces	2-9
2.9	Distortion	2-9
	2.9.1 Size distortion	2-10
	2.9.2 Profile distortion	2-10
2.10	Rules for good quality x-ray images	2-10
	References	2-11

3 Radiology devices
3-1

3.1	The basics of radiology devices	3-1
3.2	A self-rectifying x-ray generator	3-3
3.3	The difference between x-ray tubes in systems of low and high power	3-5
	References	3-6

4 Imaging systems
4-1

4.1	Introduction	4-1
4.2	Tomography	4-1
4.3	Angiographic systems	4-1
4.4	Radiography and fluoroscopy devices (R/F)	4-3
	4.4.1 Screen fluoroscopy	4-4
	4.4.2 Conventional fluoroscopy	4-4
	4.4.3 Remote controlled fluoroscopy	4-6
	4.4.4 Fluoroscopy with a flat panel	4-7
4.5	Devices for neurology	4-8
4.6	Mobile devices	4-9
	4.6.1 Mobile devices for general use	4-10
	4.6.2 Mobile devices for surgical use	4-12
4.7	Portable devices	4-13
4.8	Mammography	4-14
4.9	Photofluorography devices	4-17
4.10	Urology devices	4-18
4.11	Therapeutic x-ray devices	4-19
	References	4-21

5	**X-ray tubes**	**5-1**
5.1	Introduction	5-1
5.2	Structure and operation	5-1
	5.2.1 The cathode	5-2
	5.2.2 The focusing cup	5-2
	5.2.3 The anode	5-3
	5.2.4 Anode rotation speed	5-6
	5.2.5 The power of the tube	5-9
	5.2.6 The glass envelope and protective housing	5-9
5.3	Different types of tubes	5-11
5.4	Characteristics of the focal spot	5-13
	References	5-16

6	**The components of x-ray devices**	**6-1**
6.1	The x-ray generator	6-1
6.2	Autotransformer	6-2
6.3	The exposure switch	6-2
6.4	The x-ray contactor	6-3
6.5	The timer	6-3
6.6	The rotation circuit	6-3
6.7	Additional functions	6-4
6.8	Classification of generators	6-4
6.9	The transformer cabinet	6-6
	6.9.1 The transformation ratio	6-8
6.10	Rectification and power	6-9
	6.10.1 Self-rectification	6-9
	6.10.2 Half-wave rectification	6-10
	6.10.3 Full-wave rectification	6-10
	6.10.4 Three-phase rectifiers	6-12
	6.10.5 A three-phase system with six pulses and six rectifiers	6-12
	6.10.6 A three-phase system with twelve pulses and twelve rectifiers	6-14
6.11	High voltage cables	6-14
6.12	The radiographic tube	6-15
6.13	Electromechanical accessories	6-17
6.14	Radiographic tables	6-18
	6.14.1 Simple tilting tables	6-19
	6.14.2 Fluoroscopic tilting tables	6-20
	6.14.3 Remotely controlled tables	6-22

6.15	Tomography	6-23
	6.15.1 Tomographic systems	6-26
	6.15.2 The motor drive system	6-26
	6.15.3 The tomograph bar	6-27
	6.15.4 Turret	6-27
	6.15.5 Control cabinet	6-27
	6.15.6 Multidirectional tomograph	6-28
	References	6-28

7 Electromechanical accessories — 7-1

7.1	The wall cassette holder with an anti-scatter grid	7-1
7.2	Column tube stand	7-1
7.3	Ceiling suspensions	7-3
7.4	The spot film device	7-4
7.5	Restrictors and collimators	7-7
	7.5.1 Cylinder and cone restriction	7-8
	7.5.2 Collimators	7-9
7.6	Anti-scatter grids	7-11
	7.6.1 Grids	7-11
	7.6.2 Types of grids	7-12
	7.6.3 Grid connection and focal length	7-13
	7.6.4 Grid movement	7-13
	References	7-15

8 Automatic exposure control — 8-1

8.1	Introduction	8-1
8.2	Ionization chambers	8-2
8.3	Photoelectric systems	8-4
8.4	SSRDs	8-5
	References	8-6

9 Film changer — 9-1

9.1	Introduction	9-1
9.2	The AOT system	9-2
9.3	The PUCK system	9-3
	References	9-4

10	**Cinefluorography systems**	**10-1**
10.1	Introduction	10-1
10.2	The components of a cinefluorographic system	10-1
10.3	Radiological TV systems	10-3
	10.3.1 X-ray TV	10-4
10.4	The fluoroscopy generator	10-4
10.5	The image intensifier	10-5
	10.5.1 The glass ampoule	10-6
	10.5.2 The primary or input screen	10-6
	10.5.3 The photocathode	10-6
	10.5.4 Focusers	10-7
	10.5.5 The anode accelerator	10-7
10.6	The TV center	10-7
10.7	The TV monitor	10-9
	References	10-10
11	**Servo control**	**11-1**
11.1	Introduction	11-1
11.2	Power supply controller	11-2
11.3	Types of regulators	11-3
11.4	Servo adjustment of voltage power	11-5
11.5	Servo adjustment of high voltage applied to the tube	11-6
11.6	Servo systems for tomography	11-11
11.7	Servo-adjustment of spot film devices	11-11
11.8	Servo systems for video control	11-13
	References	11-13
12	**High frequency technique (multipulse)**	**12-1**
12.1	Introduction	12-1
12.2	How to obtain a high voltage variable frequency	12-2
12.3	A complete multipulse circuit	12-3
	References	12-6
13	**CT principles and fundamentals**	**13-1**
13.1	Introduction	13-1
13.2	A historical summary of CT	13-3
	References	13-8

14 On-screen CT

	14-1
14.1 Introduction	14-1
14.2 In comparison to conventional radiography	14-1
14.3 Concepts associated with the explored layer	14-3
14.3.1 Field of view	14-3
14.3.2 The matrix	14-3
14.3.3 The pixel	14-4
14.3.4 The voxel	14-4
14.3.5 The CT number	14-5
14.3.6 Grayscale	14-5
14.3.7 CT number scale, or Hounsfield scale	14-6
14.3.8 The window	14-7
14.3.9 Relations between parameters	14-9
14.3.10 Array size	14-9
14.3.11 Calculation of CT numbers	14-9
References	14-10

15 Principles of CT

	15-1
15.1 Introduction	15-1
15.2 Density and attenuation	15-1
15.3 Absorption of radiation	15-3
15.4 The axial irradiation procedure	15-5
15.5 The procedure for calculated attenuation coefficents	15-7
15.5.1 Algebraic procedure	15-8
15.5.2 The iterative or adaptive procedure	15-8
15.5.3 Back-projection	15-9
References	15-19

16 Mathematical analysis of convolution

	16-1
16.1 Introduction	16-1
16.2 Fourier analysis	16-3
16.3 Convolution	16-5
16.3.1 The convolution theorem	16-7
16.4 Application to CT	16-7
References	16-9

17 Forms of exploration 17-1

17.1	Introduction	17-1
17.2	Principle 1 (translation–rotation)	17-1
17.3	Principle 2 (translation–rotation)	17-3
17.4	Principle 3 (rotation–rotation)	17-4
17.5	Principle 4 (rotation–rotation)	17-5
17.6	Principle 5 (helical rotation)	17-7
17.7	Multislice helical CT	17-7
	References	17-10

18 Equipment for CT 18-1

18.1	Introduction	18-1
18.2	The table	18-2
18.3	Requirements for the table	18-2
18.4	The gantry	18-3
18.5	Requirements for the gantry	18-5
18.6	Scan speed	18-6
18.7	Radiation dose to the patient	18-6
18.8	Collimators and filters	18-7
18.9	The radiation generator and control system	18-8
	18.9.1 The x-ray tube	18-8
	18.9.2 The x-ray generators	18-8
18.10	The detection and processing system	18-9
	18.10.1 Properties of detectors	18-11
18.11	Geometric efficiency	18-13
18.12	Conversion factor	18-14
18.13	Total dose efficiency	18-14
18.14	Requirements for detection	18-15
18.15	The data acquisition system	18-16
18.16	The formation of the image in the computer	18-17
18.17	Requirements for data collection and recreation	18-19
18.18	Image display system and diagnosis	18-21
18.19	Image manipulation	18-23
18.20	Documentation of images	18-25
18.21	Recording devices	18-26
	References	18-28

19	**Image reconstruction algorithms**	**19-1**
19.1	Introduction	19-1
19.2	Topograms	19-1
19.3	Algorithms for soft tissues and bone	19-4
19.4	Coronal and sagittal reconstruction	19-4
19.5	Three-dimensional reconstruction	19-7
	References	19-7
20	**Applications of CT**	**20-1**
20.1	Introduction	20-1
20.2	Body planes	20-1
20.3	Directions	20-2
20.4	Anatomical references	20-3
20.5	An axial view of anatomy	20-5
	References	20-10
21	**The most common CT studies**	**21-1**
21.1	Introduction	21-1
21.2	Studies of the head	21-2
21.3	Studies of the thorax	21-4
21.4	Cardiac studies	21-6
21.5	Pelvic studies	21-11
	References	21-11
22	**Other specialized studies**	**22-1**
22.1	Introduction	22-1
22.2	Pelvimetry using topograms	22-1
22.3	Three-dimensional reconstruction	22-2
22.4	Densitometry of bone mineral content	22-2
22.5	Studying abdominal trauma using CT	22-3
22.6	Cerebral dynamics using xenon	22-4
22.7	CT applications in therapy	22-4
22.8	Installation of stents	22-6
	References	22-8

23 Complete tomographic installations — 23-1

23.1	Introduction	23-1
23.2	Mobile CT devices	23-2
	References	23-4

24 Digital radiography — 24-1

24.1	The development visualization with x-rays	24-1
24.2	Image scan forms	24-2
24.3	Computed radiography	24-3
	24.3.1 Advantages of CR	24-4
	24.3.2 Disadvantages of CR	24-7
24.4	Digital radiography	24-8
	24.4.1 Indirect DR	24-8
	24.4.2 Direct DR	24-9
	References	24-13

25 Mammography in three dimensions — 25-1

25.1	Justification for the method	25-1
25.2	The aims of tomosynthesis	25-2
25.3	A comparison of 2D mammography and 3D DBT	25-3
25.4	How to perform mammography	25-3
25.5	The image acquisition protocol	25-4
25.6	Compressing the breast	25-4
25.7	DBT devices	25-4
	25.7.1 Technical specifications	25-5
	25.7.2 Generator requirements	25-6
	25.7.3 X-ray tube requirements	25-6
	25.7.4 Requirements for tomosynthesis	25-7
	25.7.5 Verification testing of mammographic devices	25-7
25.8	Qualitative analysis of the image	25-7
	25.8.1 Focus calculation and measuring instruments	25-7
	25.8.2 How to use a pinhole camera	25-8
	25.8.3 Quality for diagnostics	25-8
	25.8.4 Ranges of gray in images	25-9
	25.8.5 The relation between malignancy and information in the image	25-9
25.9	Safety and radiation doses in DBT	25-9
	References	25-11

Preface

The justification of this text is the need to deliver to a wide circle of readers—biomedical engineers, engineering students, physicians, medical students, radiographers and related professionals—a basic tool to understand the basics of all aspects involved in the radiology of today.

The decision to write it arises from the proven fact that there exist almost no texts referring specifically to the technical aspects of radiology, while the literature concerning medical or diagnostics aspects in radiology are abundant. Therefore, a lot of information has been gathered to realize this work in two parts. The first deals with the basic concepts in radiology, the technique of radiographic films, the basic equipment, and a description of almost all components of the equipment used for these purposes. The second part concerns exclusively computed tomography, or CT scan. It is reviewed from the basics to the most common diagnostic applications, through the technical description of all components and elements used in the most revolutionary technique developed since the discovery of x-rays.

This book aims to give only the basics, and so many specialized items have had to be omitted, because the purpose is not to make an encyclopedia of radiology or a design manual. Consequently, we have tried to compensate for the lack of technical aspects with a concern for the didactical aspects and careful explanation of concepts, keeping in mind, as previously stated, the wide range of users.

Acknowledgement

To my family who supported me during the long period of preparation of this work, especially my son Guillermo, who contributed his talented art in the realization of the drawings, a special thanks to the companies Siemens and Philips, leaders in medical imaging technology, that provided fundamental materials for the successful completion of this book.

Author biography

Guillermo Avendaño Cervantes

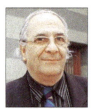
Guillermo Avendaño Cervantes is a Chilean engineer, a specialist in biomedical engineering with over 40 years of professional performance in class biomedical equipment companies and Professor at seven Universities in Latin American countries. He is the author of numerous articles and several specialist biomedical engineering books, creator of 38 innovative items of electromedical equipment, has several patents and is a member of five international scientific societies.

IOP Publishing

Technical Fundamentals of Radiology and CT

Guillermo Avendaño Cervantes

Chapter 1

The basics of x-rays

1.1 What are x-rays?

On 28 December 1895, Wilhelm C Röntgen presented his paper 'Über eine neue Art von Strahlen' ('On a New Kind of Rays') to the Würzburg Physical Medical Society [1]. These rays had been labelled with the letter 'x' to represent their unknown nature, which is understandable at a time when there was no knowledge of this strange radiation, and the nature and characteristics of radiation in general were not understood. The knowledge we have gained about x-rays belies the name, as we now possess extensive information about all aspects of x-rays.

X-rays are a form of radiation or electromagnetic wave, as are radio waves and visible light. Electromagnetic waves are variations in the amplitude of energy in time and are classified according to the speed with which they fluctuate over time. This defines the concept of the wavelength, the time taken by a wave to complete a full sequence (see figure 1.1). As a wave oscillates faster its wavelength becomes smaller and its frequency increases. More specifically, all electromagnetic waves lie in the electromagnetic spectrum, which is arranged by the wavelength or its equivalent, the frequency. X-rays lie above ultraviolet radiation, visible light and radio waves in the spectrum, and below cosmic radiation; they are a form of high energy radiation, with a high frequency and short wavelength.

We now know that the best way to produce x-rays is by accelerating electrons, which produce the desired radiation on impact with a target made of a suitable substance. This process is performed inside a vacuum tube in which two electrodes are installed. A high electric potential is applied to the electrodes to accelerate electrons from the cathode which then impact on the anode, producing x-rays. All this is possible if there is a system outside the tube controlling the process. This is similar to the conditions inside the tube of an old-fashioned TV screen, the cathode ray tube (the generation of electrons, the application of a high voltage, and the screen as the target), in which small amounts of x-rays are produced. These can be a

doi:10.1088/978-0-7503-1212-7ch1   1-1   © IOP Publishing Ltd 2016

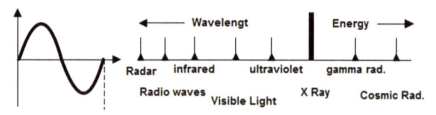

Figure 1.1. An electromagnetic wave and the electromagnetic spectrum.

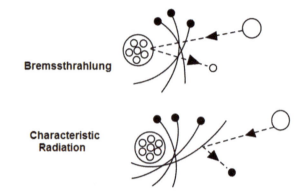

Figure 1.2. The mechanisms of bremsstrahlung and characteristic radiation.

cumulative danger to health, which is why parents are advised not to allow children to get too close to the screen when watching TV.

The exact way to produce a given quantity and quality of x-rays will be discussed later, when analyzing the x-ray tube and generators in detail. When the electrons impact the target—the anode—x-rays are produced in two main ways (figure 1.2):

(a) *Bremsstrahlung*. This form of radiation, 'braking radiation' in German, is explained by the fact that the accelerated electrons, as they hit the anode, are slowed down if they have high energy and the amount of braking (energy) is converted into different forms of radiation. This radiation is diverse and of different wavelengths because it originates from different amounts of braking.

(b) *Characteristic radiation*. This form of energy is produced by the eviction of orbital electrons through impacts with other electrons sent from the cathode, and a characteristic x-ray emission occurs for specific electron orbits.

For medical diagnosis, the x-rays typically used are composed of 70% bremsstrahlung and 30% characteristic radiation [2].

1.2 Characteristics and properties of x-rays

- X-rays are electrically neutral, that is, they do not experience deviation or deflection when inside an electric, magnetic, or combined field.
- X-rays travel in straight lines at the speed of light, a characteristic which can be used to direct and focus the rays in order to radiate the specific region of the body being studied.

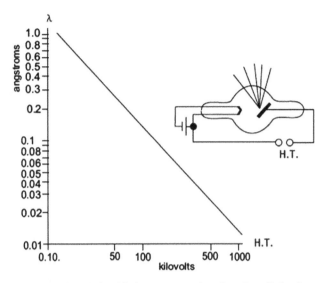

Figure 1.3. The relationship between wavelength and applied voltage.

- X-rays produce biological and chemical effects, which means they can affect an organism by producing ionization and/or cellular changes that may be responsible for disorders or further mutations.
- X-rays span a section of the electromagnetic spectrum and possess not only one frequency, but several. These depend on the set of factors that led to the generation of radiation. As shown in figure 1.3, the higher the voltage that produces the rays, the shorter the wavelength is, i.e. the frequency is higher.
- X-rays are not visible to the human eye or to animals [3], so their detection is possible only by means of instruments and photographic methods. This is an important consideration in undertaking protective measures for the human body.
- X-rays produce images on photographic film and fluorescence on certain types of crystals; both phenomena are used as a means to obtain x-rays films and fluoroscopy images on medical monitors, respectively.
- X-rays produce secondary radiation and scattered radiation, which means that a biological object receiving x-rays produces, in turn, new rays with different characteristics [4]. These rays are generally a problem in imaging and are detrimental to the safety of people who work with x-rays.

1.3 Substances and x-rays

X-rays propagate in a straight line and if any substance lies in their path they will behave according to the characteristics of the substance. In this way they can produce some of the effects already mentioned, such as fluorescence or triggering secondary radiation. Three possible interactions may occur: x-ray absorption, transmission, or dispersion. Radiology takes advantage of these phenomena to produce images, either temporary or permanent, which have diagnostic value.

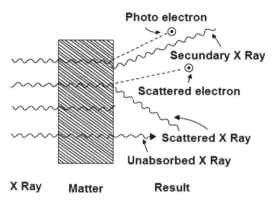

Figure 1.4. X-ray interactions with substances.

X-ray emission is obtained mainly by bombardment with high-speed electrons on targets [5] made of materials with a high atomic number. As shown in figure 1.4, the x-rays can pass through the substance without being absorbed, in which case we have transmission. If the rays do not penetrate and are stopped by the substance, we have absorption. Dispersion occurs when the x-rays pass through the substance producing secondary and scattered x-rays. The nature of the secondary x-rays depends on their energy and wavelength, as well as the substance the primary x-rays found in their way. Both types of x-rays, secondary and scattered, deviate geometrically from the initial focus of the primary x-rays, which is of great practical importance in obtaining radiographs.

1.4 The effect of x-rays on radiographic film

A fundamental use of radiation is in radiography. It is necessary to determine the penetration of x-rays in living tissue, so we can understand how both the properties of the x-rays and the characteristics of the different tissues produce a combination of effects that determines the degree of blackening of radiographic film. Simply put, the further the x-rays penetrate, the more blackening is produced. In contrast, if the radiation is absorbed by the tissue and barely reaches the film, it produces a white image. Obviously, different shades of gray are the result of intermediate values of attenuation of radiation on tissue [6]. There are basically three factors that determine the degree of blackening of the film:

(a) The physicochemical properties of the target tissue (atomic number, molecular density, etc), which determine the absorption degree of the radiation.
(b) The energy or wavelength of the x-rays, which determines whether they will penetrate more or less into the tissue.
(c) Scattered radiation impinging on the film (in addition to the main radiation) causes the deterioration of radiographic quality.

The above description is best understood by studying any radiographic film. We can see how bones are displayed in white, as little radiation passes through them,

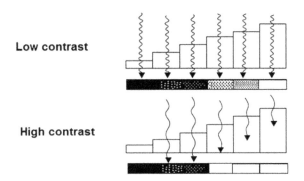

Figure 1.5. Penetration of shorter and longer wavelength x-rays and the effect on the grayscale.

while the soft tissues are black, as much more radiation passes through them and reaches the radiographic film [7]. Thus bone is described as a radiopaque tissue, soft tissues and gases are radiolucent tissues, and other tissues that provide images of different shades of gray are defined as radio-intermediate.

Regarding the above factors involved in blackening in typical practice, factor (a) cannot be altered, but factor (b) depends largely on the values selected by the technician, the voltage values and filament current [8]. Factor (c) is neutralized by various techniques which will be discussed later.

Radiation with a short wavelength and high energy has high penetrability [9], so that blackening of the film will occur if the tissue the x-rays go through is low density, producing a grayscale decreasing as the density increases, until the increase in density is such that the radiation does not pass through, resulting in white on the film. Radiation of low wavelength produces, with the same pattern of increasing densities, a grayscale that is less pronounced than in the previous case, with high densities of white and black, this is shown in figure 1.5.

References

[1] Jensen F 1995 100 years of x-rays *Medicamundi* **40** 156–70
[2] Lidio G, Lidio Y and Mosca E 2001 *Técnica Radiológica* (Buenos Aires: López Librero Editores)
[3] Mulkay J and Fernández J 1999 *Rayos X* (Havana: Pueblo y Educación)
[4] Tremolieres J 1982 *Electrónica y Medicina* vol 11 (Madrid: Paraninfo)
[5] Barroso E 1999 *Radiología de la Silla Turca* (Havana: Científico Técnica)
[6] Christensen E and Curry T 1998 *An Introduction to the Physics of Diagnostic Radiology* (Philadelphia, PA: Lea & Febiger)
[7] Vegh A 1977 Physical principles of x-ray image formation *Medicor News* **2** 47–52
[8] Degenhardt H 1983 El desarrollo de las sustancias luminiscentes y la utilización de éstas en la técnica de rayos X *Electromédica* **4** 155–8
[9] Bushong S C 2008 *Radiologic Science for Technologists: Physics, Biology, and Protection* (Maryland Heights, MO: Mosby)

IOP Publishing

Technical Fundamentals of Radiology and CT

Guillermo Avendaño Cervantes

Chapter 2

Radiographic quality

2.1 Properties of radiographic quality

The aim of a radiographic film is to show exactly what is necessary for proper diagnosis. The concept of radiographic quality considers the factors that determine the success of this aim. The quality of a radiograph depends on two photographic properties and two geometric properties [1]:
- Density and contrast (the photographic properties).
- Definition and distortion (the geometric properties).

2.1.1 Density

Density is apparent in the amount of blackening of the film, which is directly proportional to the incident radiation. A good image should have a level of blackening that clearly differentiates all structures. The densitometer is an electronic instrument that measures the density from the amount of light transmitted.

2.1.2 Contrast

Contrast arises from the existence of different densities. It measures the discrimination of two different densities in two adjoining structures. The contrast is low if two adjacent structures do not present a clear difference in grayscale. The greatest contrast is between intense black next to the brightest white possible.

2.1.3 Definition

Definition is the quality with which the details are presented, in other words the sharpness or clarity of the fine structures on the film image (or on the screen with a CCTV fluoroscopic system). The definition is affected by the occurrence of one or more of the following factors, some of which have their origin in the quality of the radiological equipment:
- Deformation through movement.
- Geometric deformation.

– Deformation from the material.
– Quantum trace.

2.1.4 Distortion

Distortion is an alteration of the real image on the film; any change, elongation, torsion, or loss of the shape in the image is considered distortion. Distortion is not always a problem in the process of taking radiographic images or the formation of TV images, because in some applications the system performs specific distortions in order to accentuate details that need to be emphasized. The magnification of a region, organ, or any other detail is a distortion, but is often sought expressly to improve the diagnostic possibilities of an image.

There are two basic distortion types in radiography:
1. Distortion of size.
2. Distortion of shape.

In the first case we consider the magnification or reduction of the actual size of the anatomical object studied, this normally occurs in TV systems. In the second case we consider the elongation or shortening of the object being studied. For example, through selecting the tube placement and patient position, image structures which normally overlap can be distinguished, and the resulting image is shortened. An example of this technique is called Towne view, in which the occipital bone (the back of the skull) is projected so that it does not overlap the facial bones and obscure injuries or fractures. However, despite the advantages of intentional distortion, devices should always be properly designed and calibrated to avoid distortion. Figure 2.1 shows how the position of the tube relative to the static patient produces shortening or elongation of the image on the film.

2.2 Quality control factors

To achieve good quality images it is necessary to control the incidence of the four properties discussed above. The quality of the equipment and the technical skill of the operator will determine the ability to control these factors. Using the

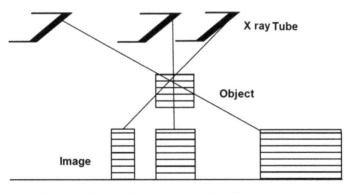

Figure 2.1. X-ray tube alignment and its effect on distortion.

radiographic technique, the operator selects the values for the generator, the positioning of the patient, the type of photographic material and the film developer used, as well as considering a range of other factors [2]. Operators have a decisive role in influencing the technical parameters of radiological devices, in particular relative to the quality of images. Therefore, the technicians who maintain and repair the equipment should be aware when an incorrect image is the result of changes in parameters and when it is the result of technical malfunction.

2.3 Density and current

The density is determined by three major technical factors:
1. The tube current or milliamps (mA).
2. The exposure time (s).
3. The product of the current and the time (mAs).

The current flowing through the tube is a result of the variation of the heat of the electron generating element, known as the filament of the tube. The current is determined by the x-ray generator, which has standardized preset current values arranged in discrete steps. The technician chooses a specific current value combined with a time value to obtain a product (mAs), which ultimately is what blackens more or less of the film. The radiographic density is directly proportional to the mAs value, so when the operator reduces the mAs value by half or doubles it, changes of 100% in the density are produced. This is clearly seen in figure 2.2. To obtain appreciable changes in the density of a radiograph, the mAs value needs to be changed by at least 25%; this is the reason why x-ray generators have selectors with time values increasing by 25%.

2.4 The relationship between current and time

There is an important relationship between the current and the exposure time in a radiograph. As the product of both is what determines a desired blackening, we can choose a combination that allows us in some cases to use a long time with a small current, and in other cases a high current with a short time. The latter can be very valuable when the need for the radiographic picture is urgent, in the case of patients

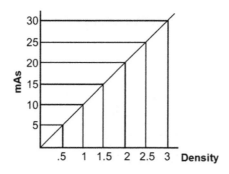

Figure 2.2. Density versus mAs value.

who are in pain and cannot be subjected to long exposure positions, and in the case of children, who often do not cooperate. Another situation where time is a consideration is the radiography of naturally mobile organs such the heart and lungs; in such cases there is a risk that the film will be affected by blurring and a lack of definition, products of the movement. In this situation the recommendation is to use as high current values and as a short time values as possible for a given kilovolt peak (kVp). Note that although we have mentioned the influence of kilovolts (kV) on density, theoretically this parameter does not control the density. However, in practice the secondary or scattered radiation (which itself depends on the kV) markedly affects the blackening of films.

2.5 Other factors affecting density

Apart from the important factors mentioned thus far, more minor factors also affect radiographic density, and must be taken into account.

2.5.1 Focus–film distance

Focus–film distance (FFD) relates to the position of the x-ray tube with respect to the film. One can easily understand that the closer the tube is to the film, the higher density is the radiation produced, i.e. a greater degree of blackening. This phenomenon is governed by the inverse square law (see figure 2.3), which says that if we alter the distance, a given density value is altered by one over the square of that value.

This can be seen numerically from a simple example: if the distance between the focus and the film is doubled, the density is reduced to one quarter; if the distance is reduced by half, the density increases by a factor of four. The equation and its application are also simple:

$$\frac{\text{mAs}_a}{\text{mAs}_b} = \frac{\text{FFD}_a^2}{\text{FFD}_b^2}.$$

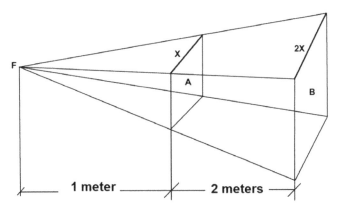

Figure 2.3. Geometric expression of the inverse square law.

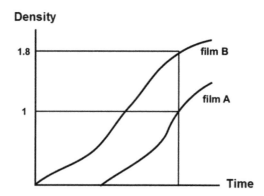

Figure 2.4. The density–time relationship for two different films.

This equation has important practical significance. If we want to control the changes in density using the current and time, we must maintain a constant distance to prevent an extra variable distorting the results.

2.5.2 Films and intensifying screens

Various related effects in films are important in determining the density. Density is directly proportional to film development time, which naturally has a saturation point. However, for a given time interval it is possible to increase the blackening of the film by prolonging the developer process. Blackening is also affected by the temperature of the developer liquids.

Reinforcing screens in the chassis or cassettes can be incorporated, consisting of special substances which through their natural luminescence produce an increase in density, as if the plate had experienced increased radiation. There are various types of screens, the fastest being those that produce the greatest density increase [3]. The same applies to radiographic films, of which there are different qualities and speeds; so that the fastest film will produce a similar density to slower films that require longer exposure times. It is necessary to consider these factors in order to suitably modify radiographic techniques. Figure 2.4 shows how film B produces a greater density than A.

2.5.3 Anti-scatter grids

Anti-scatter grids are also used to achieve a given density, and are placed between the patient and the film. These grates or grids, as they are known, eliminate secondary radiation and scattered radiation. They are manufactured in three basic types: focused, parallel and squared, as shown in figure 2.5.

The characteristics of biological tissues have a remarkable influence on the density. Pathologies and changes that cause the displacement of air at tissue interfaces are factors that affect the density. This is understandable considering that certain degenerative diseases cause a greater density on the film than structures not affected by degenerative diseases, and lungs or other organs filled with air produce a greater density on the film than those without air.

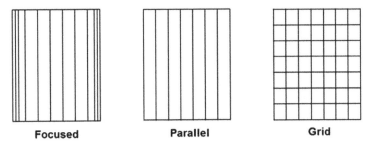

Figure 2.5. Types of anti-scatter grids.

Thus, the factors affecting the production of more or less black on the plate are numerous and diverse, so the radiologist must understand the factors that might affect the expected results. Some of the factors affecting the density can be defined mathematically, while others are defined only approximately. The mathematical factors are:
– The mAs product.
– The FFD.

The density is directly proportional to the product mAS and inversely proportional to the square of the FFD.

The second group of factors includes, in addition to those mentioned above, the voltage applied to the tube and the thickness of the patient. The radiation from the patient is approximately proportional to the fourth or fifth power of the kV used. Decreased radiation from the patient, and thus decreased density, occurs as a geometrical function: per unit thickness, either centimeters or inches, the density is reduced by the same proportion. The latter relationship is true only with homogeneous radiation, however, this is an acceptable accuracy for the practical conditions of radiology.

Based on the above considerations, a tabulation was developed and a common calculation unit was chosen for all factors influencing the density, the thickness of the patient. Each of the factors was ascribed a defined graduation, whose influence on the dose is equivalent to one centimeter thickness of the patient. The knowledge and use of this table are the subject of study of radiology technicians and are beyond the scope of this book.

2.6 Kilovolts and contrast

The main factor controlling the contrast is the voltage. The x-rays generated from high kV values cross through the tissue and impact the film thus creating varying levels of gray, thereby worsening the contrast. Lower kV values produce higher x-ray absorption of certain wavelengths, resulting in whiter regions of the film, which means improved contrast.

It is also important to note that the penetration of x-rays through the tissue depends not only on the kV value, but is also determined by the material density, the atomic number and the volume. Therefore, a kV level which indirectly considers these influences is required. The level used is between 60 kVp and 120 kVp, minimizing radiation on the patient and optimizing the radiographic contrast.

2.7 Other factors controlling the contrast

In addition to the voltage, the contrast is influenced by other factors.

2.7.1 Grids

Since the number of lead lines that the grids possess is variable, the absorption of secondary and scattered radiation will also vary. Therefore, depending on the type of grid used, a distinct effect on the contrast will be observed.

2.7.2 Collimation and restrictions

Collimators, cylinders and cones are restraining devices that limit the radiation to a specific area of the body, thereby further reducing the effect of scattered radiation that could arise in the areas covered by the restrictors. This results in an improvement of the contrast and can be checked practically when the collimator is closed while an image is observed on a TV screen; the improvement of contrast is evident.

2.7.3 Filtering

Soft radiation filters are used with the intention that they absorb specific wavelengths of radiation instead of the patient tissue. This practice has the disadvantage of contrast deterioration, because more hard radiation reaches the film resulting in a higher degree of grayscale.

2.7.4 Film

Radiographic film is manufactured to produce greater or lesser contrast. This is stated in the specifications of the film and it is up to the radiographer to select a film with the inherent contrast required.

2.7.5 Film processing

As for the density, the time and temperature of the developer influence the contrast. In this case increases of both time and temperature result in a deterioration of the contrast. Thus, in the case of non-automated developers, one must experiment with these factors to achieve optimum results.

2.7.6 Screens

The chassis known as cassettes, or chassis that do not include intensifying screens, produce less contrast than chassis containing these screens.

2.7.7 The patient

Other important factors that affect the contrast are the patient and the type of study that is being performed. For example, in some cases a cone compression is used to improve the physiological response of the pressed organ. This practice causes an increase of tissue density, requiring an increase in voltage to achieve adequate penetration, resulting in deterioration of the contrast. Moreover, certain diseases cause more scattered radiation than others: excess fluid increases secondary radiation and reduces the contrast, as in the case of pneumonia. The same applies to young children who have a greater proportion of liquid in their bodies than older children.

In short, both density and contrast are values measured by the eye of the observer. These are subjective values which are used to observe structures and organs in an objective manner, making the final task in the radiological technique a true specialism.

2.8 Definition

Previously we described the concept of definition and what types of definition losses can occur in radiographic studies. In the following sections we discuss these factors in detail.

2.8.1 Deformation by movement

This deformation is caused by voluntary or involuntary movements of the patient, which introduce image blurring. To avoid this one needs to immobilize the patient with attachments that exist for this purpose, which also provide security for the patient and allow the use of radiographic shots in the shortest possible times. Short shot duration times can be obtained using higher current values. It follows that devices with high values of tube current allow good quality images with better definition to be obtained, which is directly related to the price of the equipment.

2.8.2 Geometric deformation

Geometric deformation is commonly known as the penumbra, and should be avoided as much as possible. A factor responsible for this phenomenon is the filament (the focus), which produces electrons within the tube, specifically the size of the focus: if it is larger, more penumbra is produced [4]. If the focus size is reduced and thus the current, the operator should increase the exposure time, and then depend on patient motion control for proper definition. Figure 2.6 shows how the penumbra are produce geometrically and their relation to the size of the focus.

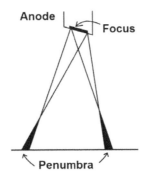

Figure 2.6. The geometric deformation, penumbra, created by the tube focus.

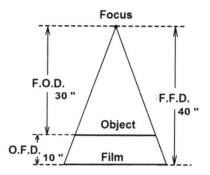

Figure 2.7. FFD and object–film distance.

2.8.3 Focus–film distance

Definition is also linked to the distance between the patient and the film: as the distance between the focus and the film grows, the definition is improved. This is limited by the projection of the structure that is to be imprinted on the film. To the extent that the x-ray tube moves away from the chassis, a cone of radiation is projected exceeding the desired volume. To avoid this, collimators are used to limit the field, reducing the influence of this factor. The standardized FFD is 101 cm (40 inches), with the exception of chest radiographs, which use a distance of 183 cm (72 inches). This allows the distance between the patient and the film to be minimized [5], as can be seen graphically by projecting the images (figure 2.7). This distance has its obvious limits, given the natural thickness of the patient's body and the chassis system that secures the holder. It is very difficult to get the film in contact with the surface of the patient.

2.8.4 The irradiated material

As well as the density and contrast effects of different thicknesses of biological tissue, the definition is also affected by the characteristics of the tissues. Thus, a thin structure can appear poorly defined if there is a high degree of secondary radiation from the use of a high voltage, resulting in darkening and poor edge sharpness.

2.8.5 Quantum traces

Also known as quantum noise, quantum traces appear on the image when an insufficient number of photons expose the film, i.e. a sparkling effect on the retina of the observer occurs [6]. This can be avoided by using a sufficient mAs related to the value of the voltage selected. Quantum traces reduce the definition because they do not provide the required number of photons to completely and clearly depict the image. This is particularly noticeable in images on a TV monitor.

2.9 Distortion

As explained above, distortion, although it can in some cases be exploited, is a disadvantage which in most circumstances must be avoided.

Technical Fundamentals of Radiology and CT

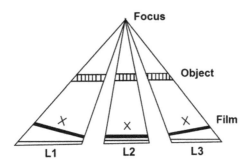

Figure 2.8. Distortion by profile.

2.9.1 Size distortion

The main causes of size distortion are a lack of parallelism between the focus and the film, as well as an excessive distance between the object to be examined and the film. This distance is also valid for the definition of the image and can be used to produce a magnification of the image, which can in some cases be useful.

2.9.2 Profile distortion

Profile distortion occurs when the image suffers an elongation or shortening as a result of a loss of perpendicularity between the x-ray and the position of the film. This phenomenon usually occurs in all radiographs. As the cone of radiation is projected, it will necessarily lose its right angle to the plane of the film. Reasonable deformation is not noticeable, nor does it affect the diagnostic value of the image. Figure 2.8 shows how perpendicularity between the film and the rays only occurs in the middle, on both sides the film has been tilted to achieve an angle of 90°, the plane shown the evident distortion.

Finally we must say that often deformations caused by patient positioning can be avoided.

2.10 Rules for good quality x-ray images

A successful radiographic result is determined by the following rules:
1. Use the appropriate mAs value and voltage [7] to obtain an appropriate density and good contrast.
2. Use a focus of the smallest possible size and a higher current value to avoid the influence of patient motion and improve the definition.
3. Use the maximum possible FFD consistent with the power of the device to obtain the best geometric resolution.
4. Use the minimum distance between the object and the film to avoid distortion of size or magnification.
5. Maintain the central beam perpendicular to the object plane and the plane of the film to prevent a deformed radiation profile.

References

[1] General Electric Medical Systems 1983 Basic x-ray theory *Training Course*

[2] General Electric 1999 How to prepare any x-ray *Technical Chart Catalog* 4863A

[3] General Electric Medical Systems 1989 A guide to radiological anatomy *Catalog*

[4] Kumakura K 1980 Improvement of x-ray image quality *Medical Review* vol 3 (Tokyo: Toshiba)

[5] Bushong S C 2008 *Radiologic Science for Technologists: Physics, Biology, and Protection* (Philadelphia, PA: Mosby)

[6] Classen F 1970 ¿Por qué tabla de exposición por puntos? *Rev. SRW* **4** 155–67

[7] Feiler M, Marhoff P and Koch R 1985 El entorno técnico de rayos X en la radiología *Electromédica* **1** 14–23

IOP Publishing

Technical Fundamentals of Radiology and CT

Guillermo Avendaño Cervantes

Chapter 3

Radiology devices

3.1 The basics of radiology devices

The basic way to produce x-rays is through the generation of electrons in a special vacuum tube. The electrons are accelerated to high speeds until they impact hard on a target, which results in the production of x-ray emission. The number of x-ray photons generated is proportional to the current (mA) flowing through the tube. The higher the current is the more electrons are accelerated toward the target and therefore more x-ray photons are produced. For this to be practicable, there must be some form of high voltage generation [1], which is the determining factor in the acceleration of electrons, and the voltage must be set appropriately for the time required in order to achieve the desired result.

Thus x-ray equipment must have, at least the, following components:

1. An x-ray tube.
2. A transformer that generates the high voltage.
3. An electronic circuit that controls the time.
4. A power supply system for the entire assembly.

The block diagram in figure 3.1 shows the minimum set of technical elements required to perform basic radiology [2]. The first x-ray devices were built using these basic components; even today, despite great technological developments and the high degree of technical sophistication of some devices, some consist solely of the basic necessary elements. Many dental, veterinary and medical systems using low power x-ray equipment are essentially a slight modernization of the first devices [3]. Contemporary electronics provide a valuable contribution to the creation of highly accurate circuits in timing, the accurate selection of values and the automation of functions, but the central idea of x-ray devices is simple and fundamental.

Most advanced devices have incorporated greater complexity. The degree of inclusion of electronics, computers and technology in general is so high that, in order

doi:10.1088/978-0-7503-1212-7ch3

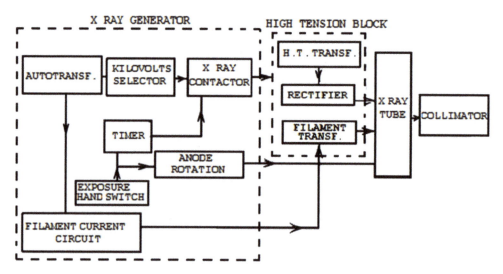

Figure 3.1. A block diagram of a basic radiological device.

to train a worker in maintenance and service [4], special courses are held in institutes annexed to the respective factories.

A basic device consists of the following elements:

1. The housing of the radiation emission system, which contains the x-ray tube and the high voltage transformer. In this unit they are enclosed in insulating oil, the small tube and the high tension transformer having a secondary connection between the electrodes of the tube, and a second transformer providing less tension but providing adequate energy to heat the filament of the electron generator. Furthermore, there may be a circuit which produces rotation of the anode in the case of a system with such a feature, and a thermal sensor for tube heating, although generally low power devices as described do not have a rotating anode.

2. An autotransformer which has triple functions: providing the voltage to the primary high voltage transformer; delivering the necessary voltage for the filament transformer to heat the filament of the tube; and also, the autotransformer can be adjusted continuously or in discrete steps using a rotary switch to control the input voltage of the entire system to compensate for variations in the mains voltage.

3. A timer circuit through which radiation is ceased at the end of the time previously selected by the operator. Radiation is initiated when an exposure switch is activated. This usually closes an electromagnetic contactor (or a solid-state electronic contactor in more modern devices) which allows one to transmit, for a selected time, the output voltage from the autotransformer to the primary high tension transformer, which is contained in the housing as described.

4. A filament circuit that takes the tension from the autotransformer, delivering this voltage to the filament transformer. This filament circuit usually has

a variable resistor that regulates the voltage that reaches the filament inside the tube and consequently the degree of production of electrons. This is ultimately the determining factor for the tube current intensity responsible for the radiographic density.

5. Other elements of x-ray devices include: supplementary circuits that produce rotation of the anode for a rotary type device; circuits to measure the radiation emitted optically and/or acoustically; measuring instruments for voltage and current; indicators for power and readiness for exposure; etc.

The block diagram of figure 3.1 shows the basic components described.

All radiological devices, from the very simple one described to the most advanced, require components for positioning the patient, such as radiographic tables, wall hangers for chest x-rays, suspended telescopic columns on the ceiling and/or walls for placing lateral x-ray tubes anywhere, etc. All this is part of a complete radiological installation.

3.2 A self-rectifying x-ray generator

As an illustrative example a of a simple x-ray device, we will explain the constituent parts and the circuit of a basic portable device for trauma applications, designed and built by the author.

The device is classified as low-power and self-rectifying [5]. The tube rectifies by itself the alternating high voltage that it receives to produce x-rays. Since the tube has two electrodes and is under a vacuum, it behaves as a diode, rectifying the voltage applied to it. For higher power applications, systems with special rectifying diodes are required [6] before applying the voltage to the x-ray tube, for reasons of performance and efficiency.

The main features of the device are:
 – A 25 mA x-ray tube with a tube voltage of 70–100 kV.
 – Control circuits with a transistorized timer and optoelectronic isolation for controlling the duration of radiation.
 – An exposure switch with optocouplers and a silicon-controlled rectifier (SCR; a thyristor).
 – The selection of three point radiographic values: voltage, current and time.
 – Dual exposure through a remote hand switch and a button on the cabinet.
 – LED supply voltage indicators, an analog instrument to measure voltage (kVp), a red LED radiation indicator, a green LED 'ready to irradiate' indicator and a yellow LED locking indicator.
 – A trolley with four wheels and a retractable support column head, with the possibility for rotation of the tube, and a height adjustment slider with positioned mechanical brakes.
 – A timer synchronized with a generator circuit, producing audio tones that change with the length of the radiation, which works as an aid to the user indicating the selected exposure time.

Technical Fundamentals of Radiology and CT

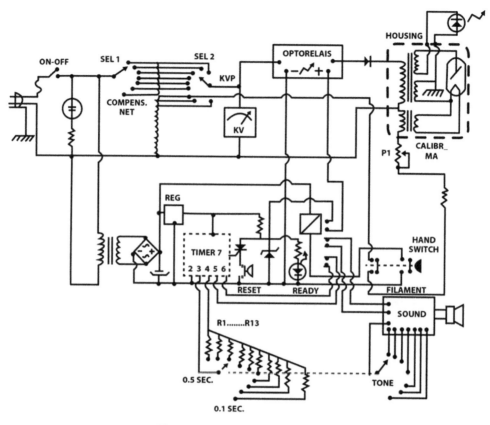

Figure 3.2. The self-rectifying device.

The electronic circuits of the equipment are shown in figures 3.2 and 3.3. The former shows the general connections including the housing (bold dashed box), which contains the x-ray tube, and the filament and high tension transformers [7].

This set-up is conventional and can be implemented in varied forms [8]. It is best to use a single control circuit based on a microcontroller that generates or regulates the times and the current level selection for the filament, allowing everything to function as necessary with high reliability and few components.

The switch SEL1, is a selector used to compensate for variations in the mains voltage with four discrete values, and the sliding contact connected to the autotransformer allows the technician to select the voltage measured by the instrument located on the cabinet (right box with KV instrument). The potentiometer P1, adjusts the filament current by providing the voltage to the primary filament transformer inside the housing. The intensity value is set to 25 mA using calibration potentiometer P1, and measured interposing an ammeter in the LED circuit located in the middle of the secondary high voltage transformer.

When the exposure shot is performed, the contactor starts the timer operation through a contact, and the LED indicator is activated. The circuit in figure 3.3 is solely for the timer, which is activated at the start of the exposure and ceases after

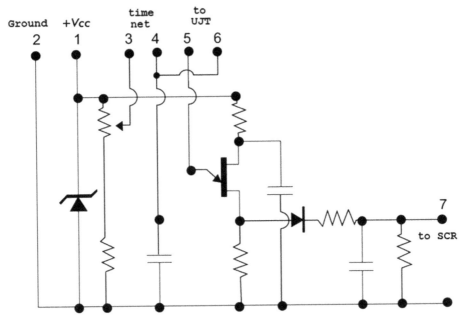

Figure 3.3. The timer circuit.

completion of the time selected by the resistances R4–R13 (connected between terminals 3 and 4 to allow the firing of the uni-junction transistor (UJT)). Closing the relay contact leads the capacitor voltage to the UJT, which triggers the chosen time after activating the thyristor (SCR), zeroing the voltage sustained by the Zener diode, so that the optoelectronic coupler opens the contactor as if the hand switch had been released, causing the end of the radiation.

3.3 The difference between x-ray tubes in systems of low and high power

Low power devices have both the tube and the high voltage transformer inside the housing, but in medium and high power devices it is impossible for the transformer to be located in the same container as the x-ray tube. It is therefore necessary to have a special block containing the high voltage transformer and the filament transformer, all within oil that is insulating and cooling [9], while the tube and rotating anode system are located within the housing. In addition, for medium and high power devices it is necessary to include in the block of high voltage four rectifier diodes that convert ac voltage into pulsating voltage rectified for better energy efficiency.

In dental devices, portable x-ray devices and some devices for use in surgery, the housing contains the tube and high voltage transformers, whereas in all other devices with higher power, the x-ray tubes and transformers are housed separately. It is necessary to connect the two using special high voltage cables [10]. All this makes the installation more complex and it requires more space to operate safely for the patient and radiographer.

References

[1] General Electric Medical Systems 1983 Introduction to radiographic equipment *Training Course*

[2] Jensen F 1995 100 years of x-rays *Medicamundi* **40** 156–70

[3] SMAM 2006 ROLLER 4 *Catalog*

[4] Billege M 1970 Mediront 125, generador de rayos X e instalaciones radiológicas fabricadas a base del mismo *Medicor News* **1** 1–14

[5] General Electric Medical systems 1983 x-ray generators *Training Course*

[6] Siemens 2007 MULTIMOBIL 5C *Service Manual* version 2.0

[7] General Electric 1983 Genetron 430 *Manual de Servicio* SM 0044

[8] Universal Allied Imaging 1999 Little Giant 30 *Instruction Manual*

[9] Carlsson C A and Carlsson G A 1996 *Basic Physics of X-ray Imaging* (Linköping: Faculty of Health Sciences, Linköping University)

[10] Jensen M and Wilhjelm J E 2006 *X-ray Imaging: Fundamentals and Planar Imaging* (Ørsted: Risø National Laboratory, Danmarks Tekniske Universitet)

IOP Publishing

Technical Fundamentals of Radiology and CT

Guillermo Avendaño Cervantes

Chapter 4

Imaging systems

4.1 Introduction

A basic radiology system is technologically simple, but in contemporary practice radiological devices that are capable of performing many different studies are required. The diagnostic possibilities of x-rays are of such importance that their applications are very diverse and large-scale; many ailments, diseases and malformations can be effectively studied using x-rays. Because of these requirements it cannot be assumed that a single type of device can be applied to any study. Although all radiological systems have common elements such as the tube and generator, different hardware, components and parts are required to create specialized systems.

4.2 Tomography

Tomography devices are used to make images in which only the regions of interest are defined, other regions, such as anterior and posterior organs on the axis of irradiation, are blurred or defocused. This is achieved by moving the tube and x-ray cassette together along the structure to be examined. The movement occurring during x-ray emission [1] has a pivotal axis on the point that is being studied, which remains static. Figure 4.1 shows a simple tomographic system, based on a table with tomographic accessories. The operation and characteristics of different types of tomography [2] will be discussed in greater detail in chapter 6.

4.3 Angiographic systems

There are imaging systems that are suitable for the study of blood vessels through the injection of contrast media [3] into the bloodstream. These devices have TV systems for observing the organ being studied during filling by the contrast medium, and also have film cameras to record the physiological process of circulation and perform the evaluation of anatomical or physiological abnormalities. Common applications are studies of the heart and large vessels, and also studies of brain circulation.

doi:10.1088/978-0-7503-1212-7ch4   4-1   © IOP Publishing Ltd 2016

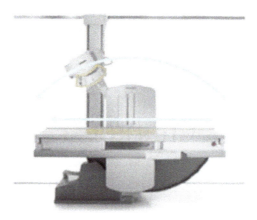

Figure 4.1. A tomography device. Courtesy of Koninklijke Philips N. V.

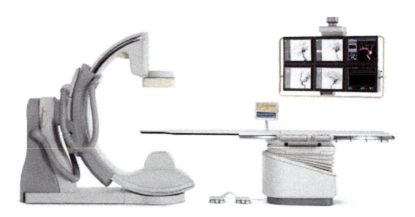

Figure 4.2. A C-arm angiographic system. Courtesy of Koninklijke Philips N. V.

This system is capable of many different motions [4] that allow its use in a variety of surgical procedures such as orthopedics, and in particular cardiology. The device has an image intensifier and an x-ray tube positioned directly opposite to each other. In this particular configuration the radiological tube and the image intensifier (or film holder) work together, generally in a C-arm or L/U-shape, with the patient's body in the middle (see figure 4.2). There are also C arms systems biplanes, as shown in figure 4.3. The system also has the ability to change from film to screen [5] and to obtain radiographs in sequence while the dye is moving through blood vessels [6].

The image intensifier [7] is a special component of the system, which allows low intensity x-rays to be amplified, resulting in a smaller dose to the patient. This allows studies with long-duration irradiation at low current values in the x-ray tube.

Image intensifiers are usually used for two purposes: (1) fluoroscopy and (2) digital subtraction angiography (DSA) [8]. Image intensifiers are set up to suit

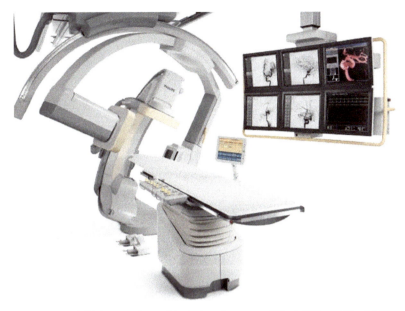

Figure 4.3. A biplane angiographic device. Courtesy of Koninklijke Philips N. V.

different user requirements, depending on the body area being imaged. In fluoroscopy [9], for example, imaging of the throat would not require the same amount of exposure as that of the abdomen [10]. In DSA, preset programs are available which enable the user to decide the rate and number of images acquired.

4.4 Radiography and fluoroscopy devices (R/F)

The technical elements that are installed for performing fluoroscopy result in a complex device which uses x-rays and produces a 'live' image feed which is displayed on a TV screen [11]. Currently, x-ray devices are the most commonly used for R/F, a combined system for applying fluoroscopy to the examination of certain patient regions [12]. One can obtain several radiographic images on the same film using an attachment called the spot film device, which lies parallel to the patient table; the latter also allows tilting and changing of the patient's position. In this spot film a set of mechanisms and electronic circuits are mobilized and divided onto the radiographic film [13], so that a series of radiographs can be documented by the radiologist of the same organ in a desired sequence or during filling with contrast. The series of images has important comparison value and can be used for the visual study of organs on a special screen or on a TV monitor. This process is performed using low level radiation (a low tube current), different to the value used in radiographic shots that are of very short duration but use more current.

Low level radiation sustained for a few minutes is known as fluoroscopy [14] and it allows the real-time observation of the anatomy of an organ or physiological function. Once a region has been located, the device proceeds to collect images on the x-ray film using shots of larger values (mA, kV, s) than those used in fluoroscopy.

There are four types of fluoroscopy:
1. Screen fluoroscopy.
2. Conventional fluoroscopy.
3. Remote controlled fluoroscopy.
4. Flat panel fluoroscopy.

4.4.1 Screen fluoroscopy

In its early stages, fluoroscopy was performed by passing x-rays through the patient, which impinged on a screen composed of special substances. These received the x-rays to produce, in response, a characteristic color. This displayed an image similar to the one obtained on radiographic film, although with less intensity and contrast. Nonetheless the image was clear enough to study the organs and choose the region to be examined. Then, after disconnecting the fluoroscopic radiation, the chassis on the spot film device was inserted between the tube and the eye of the radiologist, enabling the equipment to perform normal radiographic shots with higher values.

This form of fluoroscopy is now obsolete due to the poor image quality, and in particular due to the high level of radiation experienced by the doctor who was placed perpendicular to the rays to observe the image produced. Another disadvantage for the doctors was the need to accustom their eyes to the dark and wear red glasses to improve their vision. Also, screen fluoroscopy does not allow the analysis of an image by a group, as is currently achieved using remote TV monitors.

An example of a screen fluoroscopy device is shown in figure 4.4 with the generator on the left, the table tilted and the tube located behind it. The fluoroscopic screen scrolls vertically and horizontally thanks to the mechanical device on the right [15]. The lead protector hanging from the screen is intended to protect the genitals of the radiologist, who operates the display using the lateral handles.

4.4.2 Conventional fluoroscopy

Conventional fluoroscopy is the most commonly used system worldwide, as it surpasses previous systems and, because its application has been universalized, it also costs less than more advanced systems such as remote controlled fluoroscopy. A conventional fluoroscopy device essentially consists of an x-ray tube ('over table', OT), which normally hangs on the ceiling, and another tube called the fluoroscopic tube ('under table', UT) [16] and a spot film device on which the image intensifier is placed. This component receives the radiation passing through the patient and generates a large amount of electrons proportional to the magnitude of the radiation. This process produces a suitable image for a TV camera tube, with the advantage of requiring much less radiation than in screen fluoroscopy to obtain a useful image. This image is taken to TV monitors where it can be studied by the doctors. This method has the additional advantage of being able to use multiple monitors or a remote monitor for teaching purposes. There are other obvious advantages to this method.

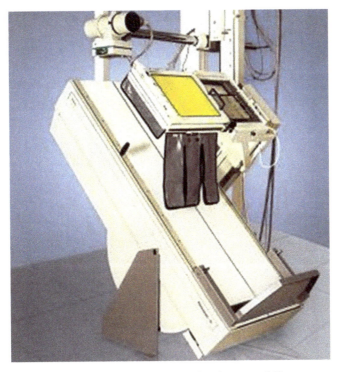

Figure 4.4. A screen fluoroscopy device. Courtesy of Siemens.

Conventional fluoroscopy is a very effective means for displaying images of the body in real time, that is, at the same time in which the events occur. Contrast media can be applied, the device is mobilized and can compress certain organs of the patient, and the table can also be tilted to allow full scanning of all regions of interest. The radiation levels are, as stated, well below those of the screen fluoroscopy and the image is superior in quality. However, as the final image is obtained after a chain of processes—the image intensifier, the TV camera, video amplifiers, optical lenses, the monitor, etc—it is likely to degrade with use and the natural imbalances of any technical system. In addition, the radiologist must be positioned to avoid being exposed to x-rays.

In figure 4.5 a typical installation of conventional fluoroscopy shows the table [17] with the tube under it (not visible in the drawing), the image intensifier mounted on the spot film device and the TV camera on the upper side of the intensifier.

This R/F system can be used for:
- Barium studies (swallows, enemas).
- Endoscopy studies (endoscopic retrograde cholangiopancreatography (ERCP)).
- Fertility studies (hysterosalpingograms (HSG)).
- Angiography studies (peripheral, central and cerebral).
- Therapeutic studies (catheter/transjugular biopsies, transjugular intrahepatic portosystemic shunts (TIPS), embolizations, stent placements).

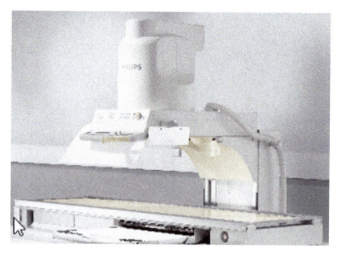

Figure 4.5. The spot film device, image intensifier and TV system of a conventional fluoroscopy device. Courtesy of Koninklijke Philips N. V.

- Cardiac studies (percutaneous transluminal coronary angioplasty (PTCA)).
- Orthopedic procedures [18] (open reduction internal fixation (ORIF), dynamic hip screws (DHS), manipulation under anesthetic (MUA), spinal work) [19].

4.4.3 Remote controlled fluoroscopy

Remote controlled fluoroscopy offers the advantage that it does not expose the operator or the doctor to scattered radiation. The device allows you to control the system from a neighboring room with the visual control afforded by leaded glass. There are two major technical differences to conventional fluoroscopy. First, there are circuits that control the operation in a remote and mechanized way, so that all movements are made without human effort. The second technical feature is that the tube is placed on the patient table, unlike in the conventional system in which a tube under the table is used.

The most obvious disadvantage of remote controlled fluoroscopy, in addition to its higher cost, is the fact that there is a high degree of scattered radiation in the room where the equipment is located, restricting staff access. This problem arises from the fact that the tube does not have the shielding provided by the table itself. Figure 4.6 shows a remote controlled fluoroscopy device. In figure 4.7 the effect of the scattered radiation produced by the tube on the patient shows the main disadvantage of remote controlled fluoroscopic systems.

Systems with remote controlled tables are currently the best diagnostic tool in the field of conventional radiology, since they combine the capabilities of a traditional table with greater safety for the operator. Also they only use one x-ray tube, over the table, so they can be used (as explained by some manufacturers) in the same way as the over table tube in conventional systems [17]. By positioning the tube with space for maneuver, images can be taken on a table or against a traditional wall hanger.

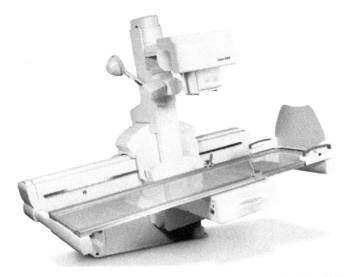

Figure 4.6. A remote controlled fluoroscopy device. Courtesy of Koninklijke Philips N. V.

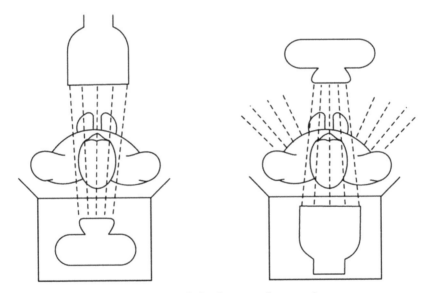

Figure 4.7. Scattered radiation in remote fluoroscopic systems.

Figures 4.8 and 4.9 show the use of a remote operated single tube device with a typical patient table and a conventional x-ray tube.

4.4.4 Fluoroscopy with a flat panel

This system is the most modern and its use is universalized despite costing more than conventional systems. The main difference of this device lies in the fact that it dispenses with the conventional TV system, the image intensifier, the spot film device and other technical elements, which are replaced by a flat panel, a high electronic

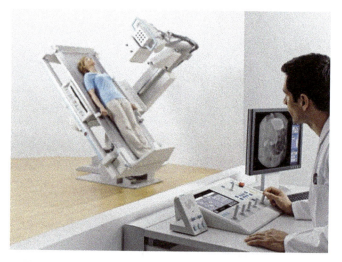

Figure 4.8. Using a remote operated table. Courtesy of Siemens.

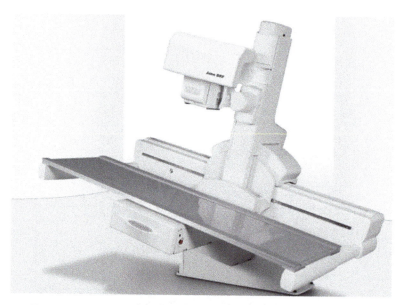

Figure 4.9. A remote operated table. Courtesy of Koninklijke Philips N. V.

integration device. This device receives radiation on one side and internally converts this into a digital electronic signal, which is sent to computers for immediate processing. Thus an image is obtained in real time and with high quality. This technology is explained in detail in chapter 24.

4.5 Devices for neurology

Specific devices are needed to carry out studies of the structure of the skull, in particular the bones of the head and certain internal parts such as the sella, the sphenoid cavity,

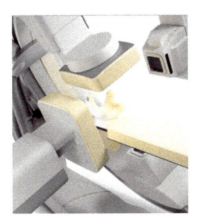

Figure 4.10. Biplane neuro x-ray system. Courtesy of Koninklijke Philips N. V.

cervical vertebrae, any kind of vascular structures, etc. The component for patient positioning and the possibility of tilting the tube make this a unique system.

This device uses similar generators to those described previously. The fundamental difference lies in the way the patient positioning is achieved. A special table is used to position the patient in any way necessary, the tube can move horizontally and vertically and swing at any angle, as shown in figure 4.10. The table is movable longitudinally and transversely, and can be moved up or down in order to position the region of interest in the most favorable way for studies of the brain (pneumoencephalography), spinal vertebrae and related studies, and intracranial surgery [18]. This device is equipped with systems for monitoring on a TV panel and the injection of contrast media. Some devices, such as that shown in figure 4.11, have a kind of saddle which can position the patient in the most complicated positions if required. The use these devices has decreased worldwide as they are being replaced by computed tomography (CT) systems, which are described in chapter 13.

Neurology and other devices can use portable film changers located perpendicular to the x-rays, regardless of the x-ray projection by the angle of the tube. These devices allow the successive (manual or automatic) firing in sequence of several film images. This allows the study of dynamic events such as the filling of coronary blood, the manifestation of an obstruction in a brain region, or the circulation in vessels of any region [20].

Film exchangers are designed to allow them to be placed under, on, or next to the patient. Some devices may be suspended directly opposite the tube and secured to it, so as to maintain perpendicularity of the film with respect to the x-rays. In other devices the film exchanger moves in a special cart that facilitates its positioning.

4.6 Mobile devices

Mobile devices can be moved to the location of the patient in circumstances where he/she cannot move or be moved; as is the case of the wounded, unconscious, those with multiple trauma, or the common occurrence of having to use the device in an operating room where it cannot be located as a stationary piece of equipment.

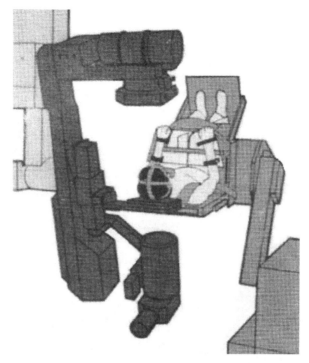

Figure 4.11. A neurology device with an image intensifier and a TV camera. Courtesy of Siemens.

Mobile devices within a health institution [21] can enter elevators, move up ramps and down aisles, and installation is immediate through wall outlets; some are motorized for easy removal. These devices can be classified into:
1. Mobile devices for general use.
2. Mobile devices for surgical use.

4.6.1 Mobile devices for general use

These devices do not have very high powers (100 kVp/100 mA) due to the limitations of volume, weight and electrical power. There is a relationship between size and the power of the system—the power cannot be increased without increasing the size of the entire system [22]. A large volume constitutes a serious obstacle to the movement of the device, in particular when being handled by nursing staff with little strength; device mobility is a parameter that is inverse to the power, see figure 4.12.

The technical parameters of mobile devices allow their use in conventional osteopulmonar applications, such as chest radiographs for classical lung studies or the determination of limb fractures. Since most urgent radiographs are included in these studies, these mobile devices are in common use in all medical locations of medium to high complexity [23].

Most mobile devices obtain their power supply via the mains of the hospital, not requiring, in most cases, special facilities to be single-phase, which is in keeping with the purpose of mobile devices, as required in two of our equipment designs, shown in figures 4.13 and 4.14. Some devices are alternately fed by the network and batteries,

Technical Fundamentals of Radiology and CT

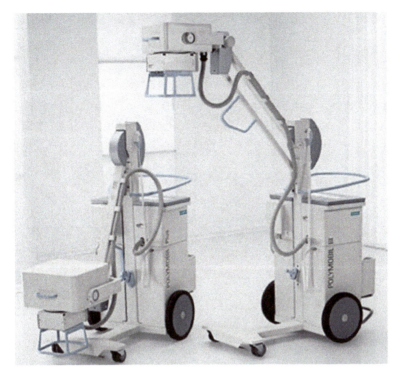

Figure 4.12. A mobile device. Courtesy of Koninklijke Philips N. V.

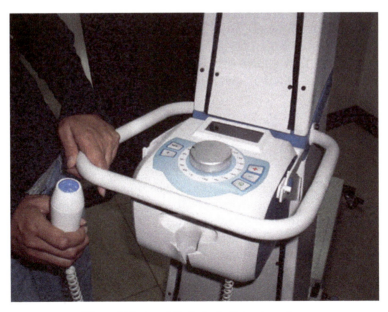

Figure 4.13. A mobile device built by the author.

4-11

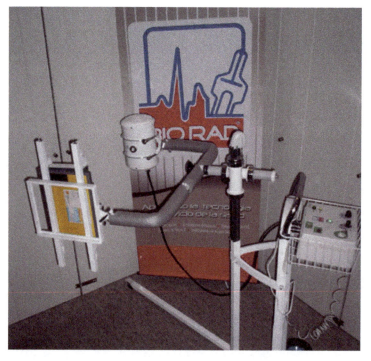

Figure 4.14. A portable device built by the author.

which allows versatility. They are supplied with a battery charger that recharges when the device is not being used.

Some devices have a mechanical arm that can support a film cassette at a suitable distance, so that x-rays can be performed without moving the patient unnecessarily. Other important additions in some mobile devices are the presence of an electric motor that allows them to move without the effort of pushing or pulling, and a special external mechanical configuration that allows easy sterilization before use.

4.6.2 Mobile devices for surgical use

Devices for surgery must have an ergonomic profile and be able move inside and outside the operating room, where they cannot remain stationary because they are used very close to the operating table, which must be free to allow surgical interventions that do not use the device. Moreover, mobile equipment is necessary in order to achieve the most favorable position for the required study.

These devices differ from the general concept of mobile devices, as they have a TV image system. They are used more in the fluoroscophic than the radiographic mode. Surgical devices are constructed with an arched C-shape in order to surround the region under study, with the tube at one end and the intensifier at the other. Their range of mobility is complete as the arch can move in all directions. The generator does not have much power so is used for longer times than other devices when

Technical Fundamentals of Radiology and CT

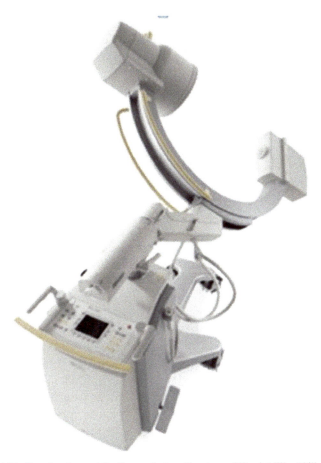

Figure 4.15. Details of a mobile C-arm device. Courtesy of Koninklijke Philips N. V.

extensive use of fluoroscopy for surgical applications (such as orthopedics or pacemaker installation) needs to be performed. A good device should have digital image storage, which can be fixed on a monitor display, while the operation is observed with another monitor in real time. This allows the analysis of images before and after interventions, or the recording of an image and simultaneous guidance through the surgical procedure without much radiation exposure for patients or surgeons.

Figure 4.15 shows a diagram of an x-ray device with a C-arm for surgery. Note that the rotating tube is contained in a block together with the high voltage transformer; these are common characteristics of low power devices.

4.7 Portable devices

Portable devices can be taken outside an institution, in order to take radiographic images of patients in their home and at sporting locations, industrial sites, military camps, or other locations where x-rays need to be taken without moving the patient. These devices are generally low power and have the unique characteristic that they can be disassembled for transport and reassembled before use. Portable devices have a limited voltage up to 90 kVp and their current usually does not exceed 30 mA. This allows the transformer and tube to be installed together in a container as a so-called monoblock.

4.8 Mammography

Mammography devices are used exclusively for the study of the female breast, primarily with the aim of distinguishing the existence of tumors, cysts, calcifications, or any other abnormalities. All mammography devices comprise a high voltage generator, a tube with a special (very small) focus, a filter, a collimator, a compression system, the plate holder with the film (or digital detector) and an automatic exposure control (AEC) system [24], as shown in figure 4.16. This particular application differs from ordinary radiological generators because x-rays of low energy need to be produced. This means using a voltage at a lower level than that used in other studies. The level of voltage is between 20 kV and 50 kV, so this type of device can only be used in this region of the body [25].

The x-ray tubes commonly used in most types of devices have a rotating anode with angled faces, where the electron generators of x-rays are emitted, opposite the cathode. Conversely, the x-ray tubes used in mammography have an anode almost without angulation with two tracks and two filaments per track, making mammographic tubes unique [26].

The anode is constructed of special alloys of molybdenum and rhodium. The voltage (kV) applied to the tube must be as uniform as possible; therefore contemporary manufacturers use special circuits from which a very flat rectified voltage is obtained almost as a continuous wave, this technique is called the frequency medium or multipulse and provides excellent images. All mammography devices should have a good system to stabilize the mains voltage supply to prevent supply voltage fluctuations from affecting the performance and reproducibility of studies.

Mammography also has a system for supporting and positioning the tube with some room for maneuver, using restrictors against secondary radiation and filters for unwanted radiation. The use of a special support for breast compression allows certain areas of the breast to be highlighted. These devices also have accessories that allow them to perform biopsies and remove tissue samples for laboratory analysis. Studies performed using mammography are one of the most important ways to make an early diagnosis of breast cancer. If the device and the technical capacity of the operator are of good quality, the images obtained show important details of tissue for early diagnosis.

The characteristic configuration of the device involves the patient being positioned in front of the device with their breast sandwiched in an arch formed by the tube on one side and the film holder device on the other, see figure 4.17. The patient needs to be under the visual supervision of the operator during the examination, so the operator should be located near the controls, protected by leaded glass that allows the position of the patient to be viewed and altered without being affected by radiation.

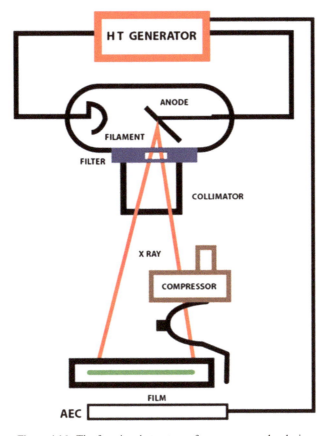

Figure 4.16. The functional structure of a mammography device.

A particular characteristic of mammography equipment is that it should have very small variations in the selected voltage, of the order of 1 kV. It should also have an x-ray tube filament with very small dimensions of the order of 0.1 mm (the focal spot) and have an anti-scatter grid with a very high density of lead sheets. The mammography device should have an AEC in order to provide better uniformity of density from patient to patient, reduce excessive irradiation and save film.

Figure 4.18 shows two examples of mammography with (right panel) the patient standing with a lead skirt to protect the genitals from secondary radiation and receiving radiation in an oblique view, and (left panel) the breast being compressed in an oblique position (note that the arc, with the tube at one end and the film holder with the compressor on the other, can rotate and take any angle). The various interchangeable compression devices, allow panoramic studies or examinations of specific breast regions.

Mammography devices are very important in the early diagnosis of breast cancer, since images of fine detail differentiate healthy tissue from cancerous tissue, and the early detection of tumor development means therapies can be more effective [27], as

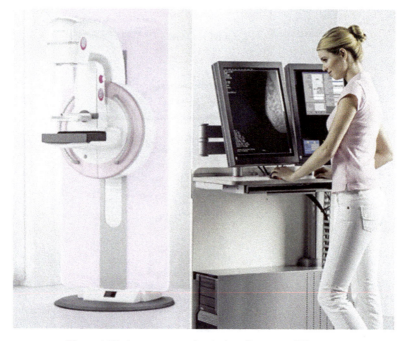

Figure 4.17. A mammography device. Courtesy of Siemens.

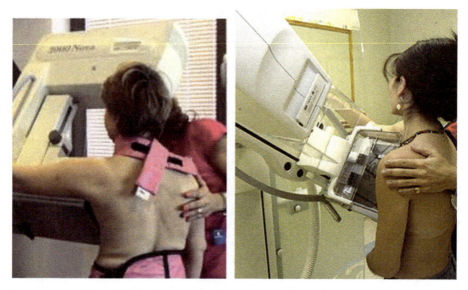

Figure 4.18. The application of mammography.

shown in figure 4.19. The existence of global campaigns for breast cancer screening has resulted in increased sales of mammography devices, both conventional and digital imaging technology, such as digital breast tomosynthesis (DBT) and 3D mammography (see chapter 25).

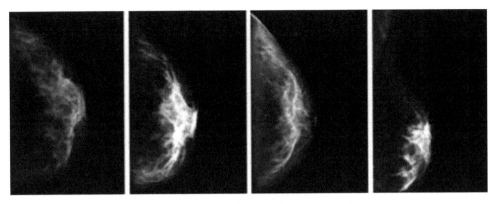

Figure 4.19. Example of images from breast studies.

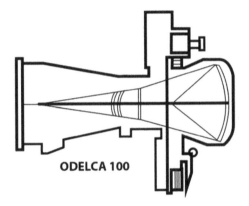

Figure 4.20. An Odelca photofluorography device.

4.9 Photofluorography devices

These devices are intended to be used in mass screenings, i.e. the study of a large population with the purpose of screening for some kind of illness [28], which can be either social, endemic, or profession-based, such as tuberculosis, sampling a population for their profile cardiopulmonary parameters, looking for silicosis or pneumoconiosis, etc.

The device comprises a module containing a fluoroscopic screen. The image on the screen is the end product of a process that starts with radiation passing through the patient, after which the image is projected onto a lens optical system and sent to the photographic film, where it leaves an image of the irradiated region.

The first devices of this type were built by companies specializing in optics, such as Odelca and Zeiss, and were used worldwide for campaigns against tuberculosis, see figure 4.20. This kind of device uses two basic systems of optical lenses [29], and documents the images in formats of 100×100 mm^2 and 110×110 mm^2,

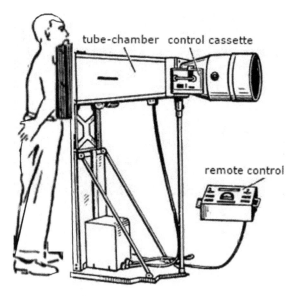

Figure 4.21. Photofluorograph.

respectively. This method allows a quick study and automatic processing of the films, and many patients can be easily positioned in a short time.

The generator for these devices is conventional, but with fewer variation levels and functions than in other applications, the main characteristics of photofluorography devices being the photographic optical system and the patient location in the cabin, as shown in figure 4.21. Some manufacturers have produced mobile systems in vehicles [30] with the object of performing studies in remote locations. This type of technology was very important in the past in the fight against tuberculosis, but is currently used less often. Modern devices are installed in shielded cabinets with special composites and use the methods of digital radiography, for example the Proscan7000 model of the Russian company Amico.

4.10 Urology devices

Urology devices are designed for the exploration of the urinary system, cystoscopic studies, transurethral surgery and physiology of urinary excretion, etc [31]. Their main feature is a tower that supports both the tilt tube holder and the table, which can be mobilized in a motorized way, from 15° Trendelenburg (a radiological position with the table tilted back below 0°) to 88° vertical. The table has shoulder supports and special attachments for patient comfort, and a support for a urinary drainage bag [32], which may be required for studies involving the filling or emptying of liquid.

The generators are conventional and the tubes of urology devices are also common to other applications [33], allowing the addition of image intensification and TV systems. There are also C arms systems biplanes, as shown in figure 4.22.

4.11 Therapeutic x-ray devices

These devices differ significantly from all those discussed so far and this difference arises from their application, since they are used not for diagnosis through film or TV images, but are used to apply radiation to certain surface regions of the body affected by pathologies that can be attacked with ionizing radiation, such as certain types of skin cancer. These devices generate soft radiation, which is achieved with units operating at the level of edge radiation using a beryllium window tube, the voltage applied is between 10 kV and 60 kV [34]. Chaoul tubes, with a conical or cylindrical anode, are also used. The device has an articulated arm supporting the tube at one end which facilitates positioning over the patient. Special filters are used in applying the therapy. The patient can be placed on special tables similar to dental chairs or on conventional radiology tables. Figure 4.23 shows a device for this application with the characteristic seat tube and the patient position, while figure 4.24 shows the dose to be applied to the thickness of tissue depending on the distance between the focus of the tube and the patient's skin. Figure 4.25 shows how different radiation penetrations according to the applied kV are achieved and the therapeutic effect in tissue layers of different wavelengths.

Finally, figure 4.26 shows how remarkable therapeutic results can be achieved with the application of x-rays in patients with superficial tumors

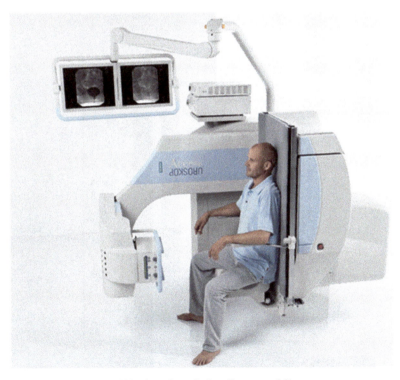

Figure 4.22. A urology device. Courtesy of Siemens.

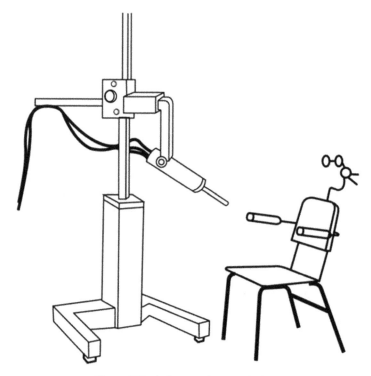

Figure 4.23. A therapeutic x-ray device.

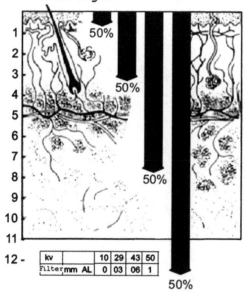

Figure 4.24. Half-values in tissue layers.

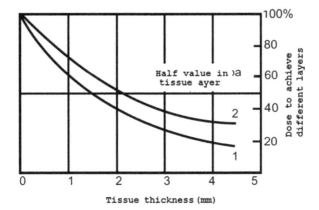

Figure 4.25. The penetration of radiation as a function of kV.

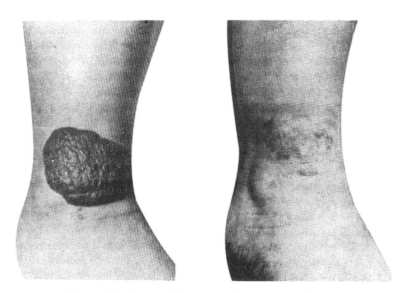

Figure 4.26. Results of the therapeutic application of x-rays.

References

[1] Finkenzeller J 1969 El multiplanigraph, un puesto de trabajo de uso múltiple *Rev. SRW* **2** 7–12
[2] Csontos M 1977 X-ray working places and equipment *Medicor News*
[3] Vittay P 1973 X-ray angiography of Medicor equipment *Medicor News*
[4] Barsai J and Horvatih P 1977 Complex angiohemodynamic laboratory systems *Medicor News* **3** 34–6

[5] General Electric Medical Systems 1985 L/U-A vascular procedures system *Product Data* B500S0B

[6] Siemens-Elema AB 1976 Angioskop *Data* MR 31

[7] Fredzell G and Warden H 1977 Kordinat Angio, unidad básica para el departamento de exploraciones especiales *Electromédica* **4** 146–8

[8] Toshiba 1999 Angio systems *Systems Data* 91623620

[9] General Electric Medical Systems 1987 L/U-angio sistema de diagnóstico vascular por imagen *Special Catalog*

[10] General Electric Medical Systems 1994 L/U-DF vascular positioner *Product Data* B5076.

[11] Biro L 1973 Development of electronic x-ray generators *Medicor News* **2** 11–5

[12] Vargha G 1973 Clinical experiences with a high reliability examination equipment *Medicor News* **2** 35–43

[13] Ness E and Heyne H 1970 Equipos radiológicos racionalizados *Rev. SRW* **1** 5–9

[14] Siemens 1974 Equipo de radiodiagnóstico estándar vertix U *Grupo de Técnica Médica Erlangen*

[15] Siemens 1975 Equipo universal para clínica y consultorio KLINOGRAPH 3 *Grupo de Técnica Médica Erlangen*

[16] Petocz J and Udvari P 1973 Experiences with the x-ray equipment of multiple field *Medicor News* **2** 44–8

[17] General Electric Medical Systems 1987 Televix remote R&F systems *Catalog* 5350

[18] Nagy E 1973 Theoretical and practical problems of traumatological x-ray working places *Medicor News* **2** 27–34

[19] Szentpeteri G 1973 X-ray exposure working place *Medicor News* **2** 49–58

[20] Szasz K 1977 X-ray working place of traumatology *Medicor News* **1** 19–29

[21] Siemens-Elema AB 1988 Mobil XR Product *Catalog* MR 81

[22] General Electric Medical Systems 1987 AMX-3 sistema móvil de rayos X *Catalog* 5349

[23] General Electric Medical Systems 1987 AMX II X ray unit *Service Manual* AO 654E

[24] Buttenberg D 1960 La mamografía *Rev. SRW* **3** 78–83

[25] Sabell M, Willgeroth F, Aichinger H and Deker J 1986 Espectros radiográficos y calidad de imagen en mamografía *Electromédica* **1** 27–9

[26] General Electric Medical Systems 1987 Mamoview mammographic system *Product Info*

[27] Biejil H 1978 Early diagnosis of mammary cancer by mammography *Medicor News* **3** 34–42

[28] Vidor T 1973 Equipment in photofluorography *Medicor News*

[29] Kovacs A 1973 Photofluorographic equipment in hospital and clinical practice *Medicor News*

[30] Szasz K 1970 Auto de rayos X para todo terreno *Medicor News* **1** 9–14

[31] General Electric Medical Systems 1989 Versatile urological image systems *Catalog* 5937

[32] Liebel-Flarsheim 1977 The Hidradjust II urological table *Catalog* AD1023

[33] Melcinor H, De Geeter P and Borde G 1982 Panurography, a new method for combined excretion and micturition urography *Medicamundi* **29** 76–80

[34] Adam G 1973 Problems of application of double anode superficial and contact therapy x-ray *Medicor News* **2** 91–8

IOP Publishing

Technical Fundamentals of Radiology and CT

Guillermo Avendaño Cervantes

Chapter 5

X-ray tubes

5.1 Introduction

The main component of any radiological device is the x-ray tube, therefore this element deserves special attention. The x-ray tube is the basis for the production of radiation and much of what can be achieved with a radiology system depends on the characteristics of the tube. The resolution, the available power and other parameters are largely determined by the construction and design of the component elements of the tube. Interestingly, despite the prodigious scientific and technical progress of recent times, current tubes have not changed significantly since 1900, when the first devices were designed with the current configuration [1].

The first device for the production of x-rays was a simple glass tube containing a vacuum and housing two basic electrodes, the anode and cathode, which is the electron producer with its respective direct heating. Coolidge subsequently invented the tube that carries his name, which was used in the first devices for medical applications. In the middle of the 20th century, tubes with the components and basic features that we know today were configured.

The main limitation that has remained over time and is considered difficult to overcome—unless a revolutionary technology appears in the future—is the energy inefficiency of the radiological tube. Excessive heat loss occurs when generating radiation; the tube receives the amount of electrical power it requires to operate and only converts 1% of the energy into radiation [2], the rest is mainly heat loss. Unfortunately, there are currently no more efficient methods to produce x-rays.

5.2 Structure and operation

The tube produces x-rays resulting from the impact of accelerated electrons on a target called the anode, the high velocity of the electrons gives them the ability to produce x-rays whenever the target possesses some special features. Electrons are produced from thermionic emission, which occurs when a wire filament spirally winding a certain length is heated by the high current flow through the wire. This filament is

doi:10.1088/978-0-7503-1212-7ch5   5-1   © IOP Publishing Ltd 2016

located in a recess (cup) contained in the cathode (or the negative electrode). When the filament is heated, electrons are released which leave the material and are concentrated in the neighborhood as a suspended cloud. The cavity housing the filament is made of nickel and has the function of focusing the electron beam.

When a high voltage is applied between the anode and cathode, on the order of tens of thousands of volts, the electrons are directed towards the anode and attracted by it. The electrons impact violently on the anode and produce intense heat at the point of collision. X-rays emerge in a shaped beam through a 'window' in the glass ampoule [3] containing the electrodes and other components of the tube.

The production process of x-rays, as just outlined, requires a set of important technological considerations: the electrode arrangement, their dimensions and, in particular, the materials, all make the construction of good x-ray tubes a technical challenge. The improvements being devised by manufacturers are aimed at achieving good heat dissipation (to protect the tube and make it more durable) and optimizing the properties and dimensions of the filaments, ultimately to improve their efficiency.

5.2.1 The cathode

A tube can have one or two filaments, according to the intended application; this filament is in the focus cavity, which in turn, is a constituent part of the cathode. The filament has a specific length, which is responsible for the power available and the radiographic resolution of the focal spot size. If the wire has more turns the focal spot is larger, and with a focal spot more power will be available, but the resolution is better with smaller filaments. This explains the fact that tubes are constructed with two filaments in respective focus cavities, this allows the selection of a suitable filament [4] to resolve the compromise between power and resolution.

Resolution is a concept related to the ability to identify fine details in images obtained with x-rays. There is higher resolution when fine lines can be seen together in the image, the opposite is true when the lines overlap to form a single spot. In short, the resolution is the ability to discriminate small details in an image.

5.2.2 The focusing cup

The focus cavity, called the cathode cup, has an important function in focusing the beam as mentioned above. The cup is electrically and physically connected to the cathode which confers a negative charge. This focuses the electrons in an orderly stream on the anode, preventing an effect called 'train tracks', which occurs when cathodes do not have focus cavities. In 'train tracks' electrons are projected onto the anode forming two lines that are detrimental to spotting very small radiographic details; the focus cavity produces a single focal circular spot [5].

Focus cavities are only necessary in tubes when high resolution is required, so they are not a universal element in all types of tube. When more power is desired from an x-ray tube, such cavities are not used because they limit the power output. Obviously the trade-off between resolution and power is resolved depending on which factor is more important in the applications for which the device is intended.

5.2.3 The anode

A key component is the target that receives the impact of the accelerated electrons. This target is called the anode and is constituted by a beveled disk at a characteristic angle. This angle is chosen such that the electrons incident upon the anode produced x-rays in a different direction to the electrons in order to obtain radiation with a defined path through a window in the glass envelope.

The technological efforts of all manufacturers are primarily focused on this component [6], because the x-rays are produced here, and the anode is responsible for dissipating the heat generated by the radiation. The anode has some important features:
- Anode angle.
- Thermal load capacity.
- Rotation speed.
- Material manufacturing.
- Electrical power.

The anode angle is crucial for the formation of the focal spot, which is also influenced by the characteristics of the filament. If the angle is increased, the area covered by the radiation beam and the size of the focal spot also increase, so the image resolution is reduced. This also creates a situation of compromise between the resolution and the radiographic area covered. Manufacturers use angles between 5° and 20° and some tubes have an anode with a double angle, one for each filament.

The angulation is used to reduce the size of the focal spot through the physical principle known as 'line focus'. This can be understood by analyzing the geometry resulting from an angular projection [7]: if the impact is on target at 45°, a resultant beam is obtained with the same dimensions, but if the angle is reduced, the resultant beam decreases relative to the size of the incident beam. Because the angles used are normally less than 45°, the resultant beam will always be smaller than the incident beam. This is clearly shown in figure 5.1.

The elevated temperature resulting from the impact of the electrons on the anode is one of the factors that limits device performance and lifetime. It is clear that the higher the temperature, the more deterioration occurs over the material, even with the possibility of producing irreversible damage to the tube. In some situations the impact point of the electrons has a temperature exceeding 1200°C. Although this is a situation of very short duration with a high peak growth temperature, the accumulation of thermal inertia does raise the temperature, so the extreme situation in which by the anode releases drops of melted metal can arise.

A limiting situation occurs when the tube temperature reaches what is known as the 'backfire' temperature, which produces a certain density of evaporated metal between the electrodes. This causes the production of a notable number of ions which convert the inter-electrode distance into a path with very low resistance. This violently collapses the system's kVp and x-ray production ceases. Therefore, it follows that the heat should be removed so that the temperature does not rise to dangerous levels. Hence there is a direct relationship between the mechanical mass of the anode and the power dissipation of the tube: a larger mass has greater ability to dissipate heat.

Technical Fundamentals of Radiology and CT

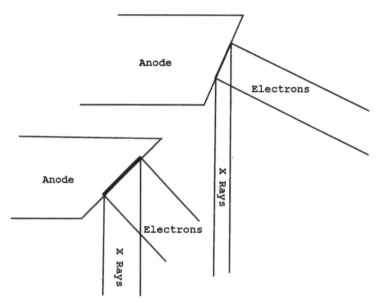

Figure 5.1. Anode angle and focal spot.

Tubes are manufactured using an anode with regulated dimensions, for example, the following possible diameters:
- 75 mm.
- 100 mm.
- 125 mm.

To measure the heat generated, 'heat units' (HU) are used. To calculate the radiographic shot in a single-phase device, one simply multiplies the kilovolt peak (kVp) by the circulating current (mA) and time (s), while for a three-phase device a factor of 1.35 is introduced in the multiplication. This simply means that in a three-phase device there is a 35% increase of power output compared to a single-phase device.

The equation described shows that a device can have a very high HU value if the tube is constructed with adequate dimensions and suitable materials. For example, if applied to a system controlled by a single-phase generator with 100 kV and an x-ray shot performed over 500 ms, using a current of 600 mA, we have:

$$HU = kVp \times mA \times s$$
$$HU = 100 \times 600 \times 0.5$$
$$HU = 30\ 000.$$

This tube has a capacity of up to 1 500 000 HU.

To work with a tube without the risk of destroying it, one must know and understand the application of two important concepts:

1. *Heat storage capacity.* This is the amount of heat that the tube can support. This concept is measured with characteristic curves called tube rating charts, which relate the kilovolts, current and time. All tubes have such a chart and

by using it properly we can determine how long the tube can be utilized in any application, considering the different radiographic values needed to conduct the study. The values chosen should be below the current curves given for each application in terms of kilovolts and time. For example, using the curves in figure 5.2, we want to perform a radiographic shot using a current of 800 mA and a voltage of 90 kVp, so we cannot exceed the time of 0.04 s. In another example we need to use a 700 mA current in a study requiring 105 kVp, this can only be allowed for a time of 0.02 s.

2. *Ratio of anode dissipation.* This is the measure of the heat that is dissipated in a given period of time; this concept can be determined by the graph known as the anode cooling curve. This graph is of great importance for the correct evaluation of the time of use of a tube. If the information contained in this curve is not taken into account, one cannot determine how long to wait before using the device again. Failure to take such a measure risks damaging x-ray studies because the performance is inadequate and moreover shortens the life of the tube. To understand the use of the cooling curve, we use some values as an example. Suppose we have the idea of performing an angiographic study that requires the following radiological technique:
   – 200 mA, 100 kVp;
   – 0.1 s;
   – 10 exposures per second; and
   – 2 passes or 20 exposures.

These data indicate that the value of the HU is 1200 × 100 × 0.1 = 12 000 HU which, when making two passes (a total of 20 exposures), gives 240 000 HU. This value is within the supported limit of the tube, which in this case is 350 000 HU, as shown in figure 5.3. However, it may be necessary to repeat the study and in that situation the tube should be left to cool for 14 min. In modern devices the computer system that controls the overall system prevents the shooting of x-rays when cooling has not been achieved.

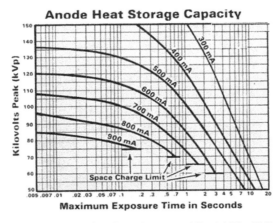

Figure 5.2. X-ray tube rating chart. Courtesy of Koninklijke Philips N. V.

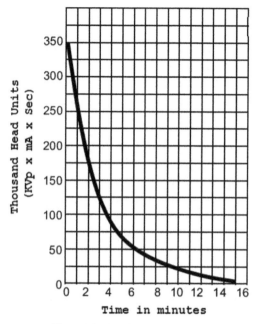

Figure 5.3. Anode cooling curves.

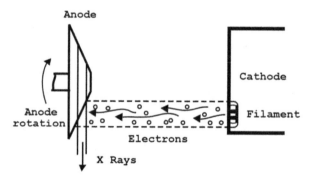

Figure 5.4. The rotating anode and flow of electrons.

5.2.4 Anode rotation speed

The speed of rotation of the anode is one of the important factors to take into account for best use of the tube. This concept originates from the fact that most tubes used in modern radiology use a so-called rotating anode, which consists of a device using the law of electromagnetic induction [8], causing rotation of the anode at high speed, like the rotor of an electric motor. The electric motor operation is based on the fact that a natural or magnetic field created by a current interacts on an electrical conductor and causes movement (see figure 5.4). Certain types of motors can move a cylinder formed by conductors, provided they are within the magnetic field and the required intensity of current is applied, as in the case of the assembly intended to move a rotary anode.

The anode is manufactured by connecting three parts: a dish that is the anode itself, a shaft that unites the components and a cylindrical block which is arranged such that it is within the magnetic field created by two external coils, which are located concentrically to the tube's glass bulb. When a voltage is applied to the coils it causes rotation of the cylinder which, in its circular movement, pulls the dish around the axis. An important feature of this phenomenon is the fact that the rotational speed is proportional to the frequency of the alternating voltage energizing the coil, this has the advantage of being able to use different frequencies for different speeds. The rotors are mounted on silver coated bearings in order to minimize friction. The high vacuum inside the glass bulb allows high speed rotation without friction with air, so special brake circuits are required when it comes to stopping the rotation after using the tube.

The electronic equipment for controlling all the functions of a radiographic system should include a special block responsible for the rotation of the tube. This, in some devices, is located in the same cabinet as the generator, while in other more powerful devices a special cabinet is required for this purpose.

The fundamental reason for use a rotating anode is that, if the anode is fixed, the impact of the accelerated electrons is on a single point. In a rotary anode, the complete region receives electrons along a track that thus shares the mechanical stress and in particular the heat. The rotation also allows heat transmission to occur more quickly, so the capacity of x-ray production of the tube increases. It follows that increasing the rotation speed increases the availability of power for the tube. Normal speeds are of the order of 3400 rpm while values of 8000–10 000 rpm are used in high speed tubes and consequently higher power is available. It is also possible to use a two-speed tube through a network frequency (50 Hz or 60 Hz), or tripling the value on the stator to 10 000 rpm, taking into account that the radius of the track has a resulting speed of 150 km h^{-1}. As a result of the higher rotational speed the tube has increased power of 70%, as the heat generated by the collision of electrons is transported so quickly and efficiently.

A key factor in the behavior of the anode is the quality of the materials utilized. The basic material is graphite, but many manufacturers use molybdenum, tungsten, copper and rhenium. The important parameters are the material's heat capacity and its ability to withstand continuous impact of electrons without significant deterioration. The pivot plate of the anode itself has a track formed by deposition of a tungsten–rhenium alloy surface. The first is critical to the production of x-rays due to its high atomic number and at the same time is an ideal support for high temperatures because of its high melting point. Introduced in recent decades in the manufacture of x-ray tubes, rhenium is a basic element for protecting the surface and thus increases the durability of the anode [9].

The need to protect the anode is explained by the fact that when turning at high speeds, the heat generated is not immediately transmitted to the lower layers and at the point of impact temperatures can be as high as 1000°C. Each surface element in a tube of 50 kW that crosses the electron beam with a focus of 1 mm remains in that area for only 25 ms. Therefore, while the top layer of the anode plate is at elevated temperatures, the material located in the lower layers barely receives heat.

This results in large temperature gradients of the order of several thousand degrees per millimeter. This enormous accumulation of heat would not be critical in itself, as the process of radiation and the cooling methods evacuate this heat, except that it causes considerable differential expansion between neighboring anodic layers. Stresses may exceed the rupture strength of the anode material and the surface can become rough and cracked.

When cracks occur, part of the electrons that reach the anode fall into the cracks and, although x-rays are generated at these points, they are useless, because local elevations retain the rays within the anode. Approximately half of the electrons disappear inside the cracks, which means that half of the tube current is lost in the cracks. A tube of 50 kW which has aged thus has an output which is no greater than that of a tube of 25 kW. The pure tungsten disadvantage of cracking well below melting temperatures must be compensated by a lower load at the specific point of impact, therefore, including 10% of rhenium alloy can significantly extend the life of the tube.

In short, we can say that an anode has a tungsten–rhenium alloy as a surface layer with a thick layer of molybdenum below. The graph in figure 5.5 shows the effects described.

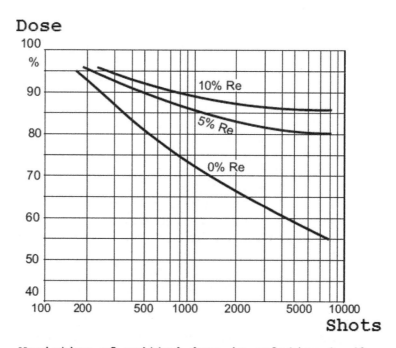

Variation of emitted dose in relation to the number of shots X Ray and with the proportion of Rhenium in alloy Tungten

Figure 5.5. The effect of rhenium as a percentage of alloy anodes.

5.2.5 The power of the tube

This concept is related to the characteristics of the anode. As the size of the anode surface increases so does the power, this is due to the fact that the power is directly related to the circulating current, which is a direct function of the number of electrons, which in turn is determined by the surface area of impact. The larger this area is the more electrons are incident thereon and more x-rays can be produced.

Power is measured by multiplying the current by the voltage applied between the electrodes, according to the following expression:

$$Power(kW) = mA \times kVp/1000.$$

It should be remembered that the power is related to the dimension of the focal spot (higher output current) and to the anode angle; a smaller angle increases the power. Moreover, the rotational speed of the anode is directly proportional to the power, as discussed above.

In short we can say that power depends on:
1. The size of the anode; a larger anode is more powerful.
2. The size of the focal spot; more power is produced at a larger focal spot.
3. The anode angle; a larger angle leads to lower power.
4. The rotation speed; the power is greater at higher speeds.

The powers one can obtain with x-ray tubes cover a wide range level of possibilities: 12, 15, 19, 22, 24, 27, 30, 37, 40, 43, 50, 58, 65, 70, 75, 76, 85, 100, 125, 130 and 140 kW. Different values can be obtained for the same tube at different rotational speeds, for example a 37/65 tube with a focus of 1.5 mm has 37 kW power at a speed of 3400 rpm and 65 kW at 10 000 rpm. The most commonly used values for the anodic angle are: 6.5°, 10°, 11°, 12°, 12.4°, 15°, 16° and 20°. The best use of a tube is achieved by considering the interrelationship of these factors on charts that specify the characteristics of the focal spot, speed, power output and anode angle.

Finally, in most x-ray devices with computerized generators, optimal utilization is controlled through automated calculation of the parameters of the installed tube. There are also circuits that monitor prohibited conditions and prevent the x-ray shot if values exceeding the specifications are applied to the tube.

5.2.6 The glass envelope and protective housing

The tube also has a glass envelope which contains all the elements discussed. The envelope is known as a bulb and is made from a special type of glass (Pyrex), which is chosen for its properties of high mechanical and tensile strength, and in particular for its thermal resistance. The inner surface of the casing tube is designed for the filtration of rays on the entire surface except in the region known as the window, which is less thick and has no x-ray shield, allowing the x-rays to exit the window outwards. Once the components have been placed in the tube, a high vacuum is applied in order to obtain complete evacuation of air, thus preventing oxidation and the possibility of the high voltage being altered.

The metallic tube support consists of materials that are strain resistant and have the function of supporting and protecting the tube. The support contains a special oil intended to facilitate cooling and isolation of the tube. Some tubes have a circulation system and a radiator that moves and cools the oil so that continued use can be made of the tube without heat build-up and damage. Such elements are common in the tubes used in fluoroscopy and CT.

There are basically three ways to support the high tension cables according to the angle at which the cables are connected to the tube: supports with angles of 0°, 180° and 90° between the window of the tube and the cables.

Figure 5.6 depicts a typical x-ray tube showing the different constituents in detail without the metallic housing, i.e. only the bulb with its internal elements. The left side shows the cathode connection with the feeding points of the filament.

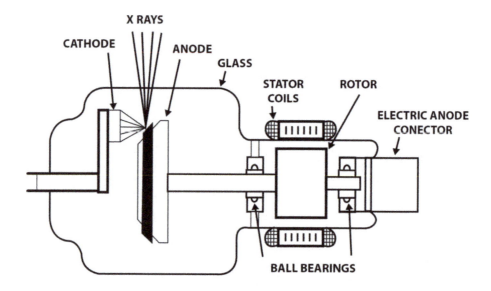

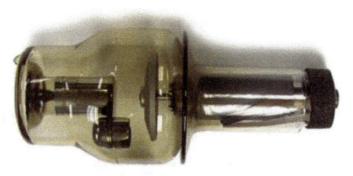

Figure 5.6. Components of an x-ray tube.

5.3 Different types of tubes

Based on the specific application, we have the following classification of x-ray tubes:
1. Normal x-ray tubes.
2. Fluoroscopic and radiographic tubes.
3. Cineradiography tubes.
4. CT tubes.
5. Mammographic tubes.
6. Tubes for therapy.

The first two types do not differ in shape, power or construction, the difference is mainly in the form of support and cooling applied, although some manufacturers use the same type of tube for both applications. Cineradiography tubes have a specific difference, a grid which receives a negative voltage for control of the emission of electrons during short periods of time; this gives the possibility of pulsed cine. Therapy tubes have a different construction, since their purpose is to generate x-rays of different energies than those applied in diagnostic radiology. Mammographic tubes have a special small filament and a different location for the rotating anode.

Tubes for cineradiography have a third electrode (called the control grid) for switching or manipulating the transfer of electrons from the cathode to the anode. A negative potential of appropriate magnitude (about 3000–4000 V) applied for some time (2–5 ms) allows the exit of electrons to be blocked instantly. The tubes that have this type of grid allow control radiographic exposures up to a frequency higher than 150 s^{-1}.

It should be noted that the control grid is different in function from the focusing cup. The focusing cup is used in all kinds of tubes. Its negative polarity is the result of its attachment to the cathode. The cup is at the end of the cathode and contains the filament which emits electrons, the effect is the focusing of the electron beam. This beam has a conical projection that travels towards the anode, produced by the focuser effect of the electro-negativity in the cup, as shown in figure 5.7.

The operation of CT tubes is not different from conventional tubes, but they are designed and constructed to withstand the rigorous conditions of use to which they are subjected. Mammographic tubes have some different characteristics located in the filament and anode. Mammography tubes are unique, because not only do they differ in terms of the fineness of the filament with respect to other tubes, they also differ in terms of their anode. Most x-ray tubes have an angled rotating anode that faces the cathode where electrons are emitted. The tubes used in mammography [10] have almost no angle to the anode, instead they have tracks (one made of molybdenum and the other made of rhodium) and two filaments per track (see figure 5.8). Anode–filter combinations are used and are manufactured as molybdenum–molybdenum or molybdenum–rhodium.

In terms of anode rotation there are two types of tube:
1. Rotating anode tubes.
2. Tubes with a fixed anode.

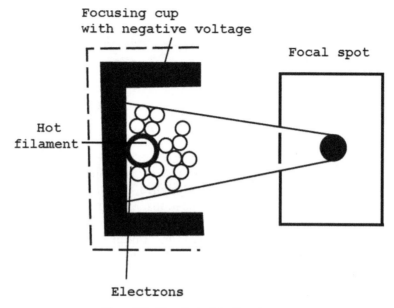

Figure 5.7. The effect of the focusing cup.

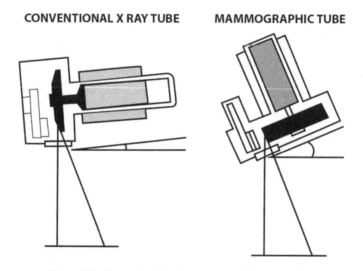

Figure 5.8. Conventional and mammographic x-ray tubes.

The first has already been studied in detail. Fixed anodes have a special structure.

Stationary anode tubes are constructed with a tungsten film implanted on a thick copper cylinder, which is a better conductor of heat than tungsten; through this, mass dissipation of the heat produced can be achieved. The fixed anode has an angle which can vary between 15° and 20°, allowing good coverage to be achieved but with poor resolution. This is explained by the fact that, by not having a rotating anode, it is necessary for the focal spot to be larger to obtain adequate power. These types of tube use only one filament and have limited practical applications. At present their use is restricted to certain mobile devices, dental radiology devices, some low power devices for emergency radiography and x-ray therapy.

Finally, we mention the existence of a different type of tube, which produces electrons through high-field emission. This does not require a filament, so it is known as a cold cathode or high-field emission tube. In these tubes the cathode surrounds the conical anode.

5.4 Characteristics of the focal spot

As discussed above, the focal spot and size of the filament are important in relation to the desired resolution and power. Reducing the focal spot improves the ability to distinguish small details, i.e. the resolution improves. However, at the same time the power is reduced.

There are two types of focal spot, the actual focal spot and the effective focal spot, both are defined in terms of functions of the angular projection obtained from the angled anode. The effective focal spot size is the resulting beam of radiation leaving the anode bezel, while the actual focal spot is the size of the electronic beam impacting on the bezel. Obviously, the value that really matters is the effective focal spot, as this is the amount of radiation that goes outside the tube. This value is found in manufacturer specifications.

Since the focal spot results in a compromise between power output, resolution and exposure time, it is not possible to obtain the smallest focal spot size, highest power and shortest exposure time simultaneously. Other factors affecting the size of the focal spot are the wire diameter of the tungsten filament, the number of turns of the filament, the voltage applied between the electrodes and the milliamps of current produced. Thus, the focal spot is amplified by increasing the number of filament turns, its diameter and current, which is explained by the fact that the production of electrons is greater and the greater density of these increases the size of the focal spot. Increasing the kVp produces a thin electron beam, reducing the size of the focal spot.

To measure the focal spot two methods are used [11]:

1. *Camera hole or pin hole.* This method is used when focal spots larger than 0.3 mm are to be measured. The camera is connected to the output window of the tube, which has a small hole drilled in it on a thin gold foil in the middle of the structure. On the opposite side of the chamber is a cavity containing dental radiographic film. The fine hole produces an inversion of the optical radiation beam which strikes the film, producing an image proportional to the focal spot size. The whole measurement process can be seen clearly in figure 5.9.
2. *The star test.* An instrument (called the star pattern) projects a star pattern in the beam (see figure 5.10). The merging of the smaller lines in the image shows the degree of resolution obtained, which is proportional to the size of the focal spot.

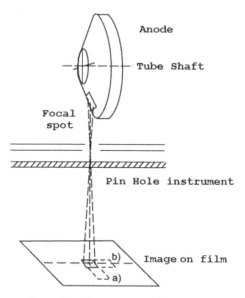

Figure 5.9. Measurement with a pin hole.

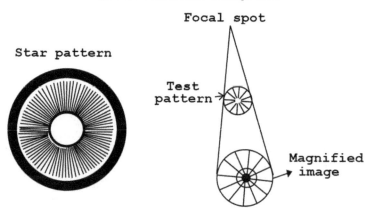

Figure 5.10. The star pattern. Courtesy of General Electric.

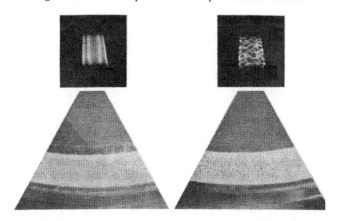

Figure 5.11. The effect of using the anode track. The figure on the right shows a damaged anode surface. Courtesy of Siemens.

Technical Fundamentals of Radiology and CT

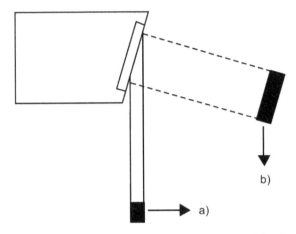

Figure 5.12. (a) The effective focal spot and (b) the actual focal spot.

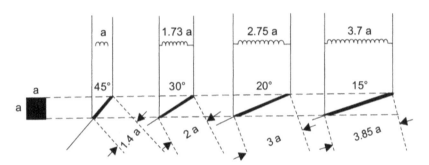

Figure 5.13. The relationship between anode focal spot and angle.

The pin hole is also used to obtain an image that shows the effect of using the anode track, as shown in figure 5.11. This can be used to locate a damaged track, as it produces a grainy picture on the photographic plate. In figure 5.11 a comparison is made between a damaged track and a little-used track; this gives a direct snapshot of the state of the anode.

The actual focal spot is also called the heat reservoir, because it is actually impacting on the region where the electrons release heat, while the effective focus is also called the optical focus because it is the one that produces the projection of radiation. This is clearly shown in figure 5.12.

When the anode was discussed, we said that the focus is determined by the inclination of the anode. This is shown in figure 5.13, which demonstrates the fact that the same product ($a \times a$) can be achieved with different anode angles, so dissipation can be obtained with a small focal spot. We can see that a smaller angle determines that the anode achieves a smaller focal spot (for the angle) and at the same time good heat dissipation, such that a tube can have good dissipation for a small effective focal spot and high energy radiation for a large actual focal spot.

References

[1] General Electric Medical Systems 1983 X-ray tubes *Training Course*

[2] Universal X-ray Inc 1988 UX tube *Engineering Info Operation Manual* 105

[3] Universal X-ray Inc 1988 Instruction for assemblers and users *Engineering Info* 116

[4] Philips 1986 Super Rotalix, high performance rotating anode tubes for 125 kV and 150 kV *Product Data* SFX 66

[5] General Electric Medical Systems 1997 X-ray tube unit evacuating and oil filing system *Direction* SP-1568A

[6] Universal X-ray Inc 1988 Seasoning of tubes *Engineering Info* 111

[7] Geldner E 1982 Nueva redacción de la norma sobre focos de tubos de rayos X *Publicación de IEC* 336/81

[8] Appelt G and Dietz H 1978 An upper limitation of output in rotating anode X ray tubes *Electromedica* **3** 76–80

[9] Universal X-ray Inc UX technical data UX-51H-41M 1987 *Engineering Info* 09-29

[10] Wilson Ch R 2010 *Review of the Physics of Mammography* (Milwaukee, WI: Medical College of Wisconsin)

[11] Sutherland W H 1982 Mediciones del foco con la cámara de orificio en los tubos de terapia *Electromédica* **2** 45–9

IOP Publishing

Technical Fundamentals of Radiology and CT

Guillermo Avendaño Cervantes

Chapter 6

The components of x-ray devices

6.1 The x-ray generator

The main device in any radiological system is the x-ray generator, which consists of a metallic cabinet containing a set of electrical and electronic components. This device allows the operator to select the values and parameters required to achieve images using x-rays or dynamic images using the fluoroscopic mode, for purposes of diagnosis.

All generators contain the necessary elements to create signals and send instructions to the x-ray tube in order to emit radiation of the specified amount and necessary duration. These components allow the selection of the voltage to be applied to the tube, the current flow through the tube, the value of current flowing through the filament (which will determine how much x-ray emission will be produced [1]) and also how long the radiation will last. In the case of an installation with more than one tube, the components allow the operator to select which tube to use and also which filament will be used if the tube has more than one filament. The operator can choose whether the films will be used with or without an anti-scatter grid and also select other factors necessary to obtain the best functioning of the whole radiological installation.

Figure 6.1 shows the overall scheme of an x-ray system where the generator (enclosed in the rectangle on the left side) shows the fundamental components contained therein. From the generator [2], the electric signals go to the high voltage transformer cabinet, inside which are located rectifiers for the high tension and the filament transformers; other electric signals from the generator are destined to control anode rotation in the tube.

The choice of values by the operator occurs in the generator [3], which has selectors where the number of kilovolts is determined, modifying the voltage of the power supply transformer, and the preset values of current filament and exposure time are also selected.

doi:10.1088/978-0-7503-1212-7ch6   © IOP Publishing Ltd 2016

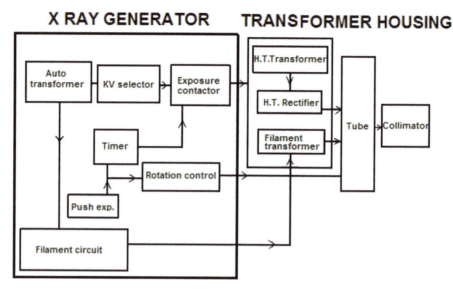

Figure 6.1. A diagram of a complete radiology system.

6.2 Autotransformer

The design of an x-ray generator starts with an autotransformer [4] which is connected to the electric network from the primary side, which usually has several taps, so that a selector connected to these taps compensates the fluctuation in the voltage supply. Several other taps are available on the secondary side of the autotransformer, which allow different voltages to be generated from them. Different values of kilovolts can be applied on the tube by the high voltage transformer which is fed with a single voltage at a time. This is selected from the different values available on the taps and the selection is made by the operator who choses according to the penetration depth desired.

From the autotransformer, voltages are taken to feed the filament transformer which heats the filaments with variable voltages to achieve different amounts of x-ray emission. As all tubes require a process of thermo-ionic electron generation, it is a fundamental requirement to have a circuit that can establish and allow adjustment of the current of the filaments. This circuit is of great importance since the accuracy of the heating current values determines the accuracy of the current flow for each shot. This is so significant that one of the tasks of radiographic calibration [5], which is performed by the technical staff, is the adjustment of the filament heating current.

6.3 The exposure switch

All x-ray units have an exposure push button operated by the technician who initiates the production of radiation. Most manufacturers design this device to work in two successive steps. When it is activated at the first step the rotation of the tube starts along with increased tension filament heating. The filament is pre-heated to a value which is inadequate to generate x-rays of good quality, but necessary to avoid starting the filament heating from a zero level each time so that it is necessary to use the switch to take a radiographic shot. This increased heating condition, obtained with the push button, is called the 'booster' and is critical to the quality of radiography. When the second step of the exposure push button is applied, the x-ray contactor and the timer are activate simultaneously, so the operator holding the activated switch expects that the timer will cut the radiation, disconnecting the contactor before the operator completes their manual action.

6.4 The x-ray contactor

The contactor is the technical element that applies the selected voltage from the autotransformer to the primary side of the high voltage transformer. This phenomenon occurs only during the shooting time determined by the timer. The x-ray contactor is basically a switch controlled by an electromagnet that closes and then disconnects when the timer gives the order, opening the electric connection and ceasing radiation. The first devices used an electromagnetic contactor, however, the solid-state contactors currently used have a longer life and are also preferred because they do not wear out the pattern of each contact, nor are they affected by sparks arising from connecting and disconnecting, and, in addition, they are noiseless.

6.5 The timer

The choice of radiation time is also carried out in the generator; as already mentioned this task is entrusted to the timer. There are different ways to design and build timers and all have as a requirement not only the proper calibration of values, but also the recording of the same. This is particularly important in terms of reliability and it is obvious that for an equal duration of shooting the results obtained should be the same. Timers have a variety of values of exposure duration to select and are designed based on solid-state circuitry. When the contactor is activated x-ray radiation is initiated and when the selected time is reached, the timer disconnects the x-ray contactor and stops the radiation.

6.6 The rotation circuit

In most devices the generator is responsible for providing the supply voltage to start the rotation of the tube and maintain it during the shooting time. Thereafter, a special circuit is used that is responsible for providing an opposite voltage, used to brake the rotation once shooting has taken place. In some cases the rotation is created by special circuits which are physically located outside the generator, for example high speed anode starters.

We know the reason for the rotation of the tube, what matters now is how to rationally use the rotation. First it must be noted that the tube will wear out its ball bearings the more rotations that are made; this is why the operator of the equipment must enable the shortest time possible for the rotation mechanism to start when the push button is used in the first step. The braking mechanism for the rotation is also designed to maintain the ball bearings.

Moreover, in almost all devices, there is a circuit for blocking the radiographic shot if the anode is not rotating, due to flaws in the tube itself or faults in the rotation circuit. This is done in order to prevent the impact of the accelerated electrons on only one point of the anode track and consequently destruction of the tube. These consequences can arise in some devices if failures occur in the blocking circuit and the shot is permitted without rotation.

Finally, we look at the case where the rotation circuits [6] have a high starting voltage in order to overcome the inertia of the rotating anode. Once the required speed has been reached, a timed circuit connects the rotating anode to a lower sustaining voltage that is responsible for maintaining the rotation until the end of the shot.

6.7 Additional functions

Basic devices comprising the components mentioned above exist in many conventional radiological facilities, however, there are larger installations that require other complementary functions. Among the most commonly used are the switching circuits of work stations, in which the generator can be enabled to control the function of two or more tubes. A further function that is widely used is the switching of both foci inside the same tube; the trade-off between resolution and power requirements determine the choice of one or the other. Another function may be the use of an automatic x-ray dose control [7], which aims to control the duration of a shot automatically, cutting radiation when the desired values have been reached. These functions and how to implement this system will be studied later.

Some devices are equipped with circuits and components designed to perform tomograms; the selection of this function is also located in the generator. Another function is the selection of a radiological TV system, which allows the fluoroscopic observation of the regions or organs that are being explored before use of x-ray exposures. This possibility of switching between modes is located on the generator. Also located on the generator is the selector for table or wall anti-scatter (Bucky), which are required for a diverse range of radiographic studies [8]. This device will be discussed in detail below.

Some special buttons for remote controlled tables allow one to make a selection of the exposure parameters already studied [9], while also controlling the movements of the table, the abdominal compressor, patient movements, spot film function, the angle of the tube, opening or closing of collimators, etc.

6.8 Classification of generators

Much of what is obtained in a radiographic study is determined by the generator, so it is one of the vital components of an installation and, not surprisingly, they have evolved in terms of technological development. This allows us to make a qualitative classification of the generators as follows.

    1. In electromechanical generators, the use of selectors, switches and relays predominates, together with resistors and transformers. Another important feature is the use of valve-type rectifiers (vacuum or gas). These instruments are of the galvanometer type (a needle on a scale). In these first-generation devices the generator and mechanical timers are simple but reliable long-life circuits.

2. Second-generation generators include the use of electronic circuits (mainly vacuum valves) for timers, switching functions, automatic network stabilization, rotation of the tube and measuring parameters. The firing of the x-ray is performed, as in the previous type, through power relays. Complex rectification systems are designed (polyphase) in order to obtain more uniform shooting voltages. An important improvement comes with the addition of solid-state high voltage rectifiers, which lengthen the life of high voltage systems and reduce their size. This type of device has better operation of the equipment and tube, with a constancy and repeatability of the selected radiographic values, but has the major disadvantage of a much higher failure rate than first-generation devices. This is mainly due to the incorporation of a larger number of components, which increases the failure rate.
3. In third-generation devices a higher level of integration of electronic components is incorporated, which allows more accurate calibration, new protective circuit blockers or prohibition using the tube characteristics values and, in particular, a novel firing system obtained through semiconductors (thyristors) that eliminates the use of relays (which wear out the moving parts and the parts that are hit at each shot). The quality and variety of studies is higher in these devices, in particular with regard to the possibility of repeating a technique accurately. These devices have proven to have the lowest reliability of all types, due in part to the large number of circuits, which increases the failure rate.
4. Fourth-generation devices incorporate computing circuits (see figure 6.2), in particular microprocessors, to perform all the controls and functions of the generator much more reliably and accurately. This reduces the size of the generator dramatically while still achieving the required powers. This is the most up-to-date generation of devices, but obviously new manufacturing technologies (fiber optics, surface mount components, liquid crystal displays or plasma displays, etc) are constantly being incorporated. Devices of this generation include components made using the technique of medium frequency (higher than the network which is 50 Hz or 60 Hz), which originate from ingenious systems of solid-state switching. These circuits

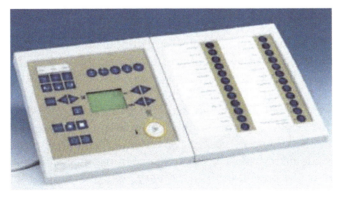

Figure 6.2. A fourth-generation generator. Courtesy of Siemens.

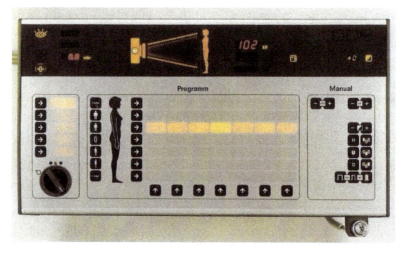

Figure 6.3. An x-ray generator. Courtesy of Siemens.

give rise to multi-pulse generators (or high frequency generators) as shown in figure 6.3, which increase the high voltage performance, significantly reducing the size of the voltage step-up transformers and eliminating some components using high voltage cables, and significantly improve the energy efficiency of the radiation to achieve more continuous emission over time, similar to having an applied voltage of direct current in the tube.

6.9 The transformer cabinet

The component responsible for supplying the high voltage to the tube is the high voltage transformer. This is contained in a robust cabinet which also holds the electronic components for rectifying the alternating voltage in order to apply a continuous voltage between the anode and cathode of the tube.

The following components are included in the transformer cabinet:
- The high voltage transformer.
- The filament transformer.
- The rectifiers.
- The switch to select the x-ray tubes.
- The switch to select the filaments (large or small).
- The terminal strip for connection to the generator.
- The female connectors for the high tension cables.

As the power becomes higher, the size of the transformers grows in addition to changes to the rectification system and the conformation of the transformer. There are some configuration differences between single-phase and three-phase transformers. As in any conventional transformer, high voltage transformers also have primary and secondary sides; in the present case the primary voltage is supplied by the generator and reaches the cabinet high voltage via interconnect cables, while the secondary side

Technical Fundamentals of Radiology and CT

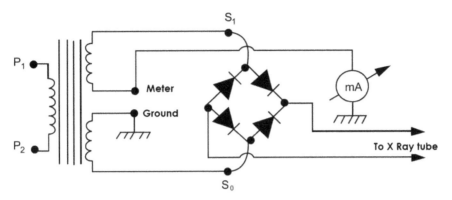

Figure 6.4. A high voltage transformer circuit diagram.

has the more specific features. Any type of x-ray transformer should possess a secondary with many turns to achieve the desired high voltage. This means that the number of windings per layer is very high, with the consequent inconvenience of a very high voltage between layers, so they must be constructed with special insulation polyesters or oiled paper between them. In the design of high voltage transformers for radiological use, it is customary to divide the secondary into two coils, installing between both coils the ammeter that measures the tube current (mA), with one terminal grounded, as shown in figure 6.4.

Another feature of the secondary side is the high impedance facing the coils. Such resistance values and reactance cause a voltage drop that is included in the circuit of the output current, hence the need to find a compromise between the number of turns and their size. Secondary coils are separated into two parts, electrically connected so that one is connected to the ammeter to measure the circulating current. The other similar coil is connected at one end to one point of the rectifier and at the other end to the output of the same instrument, the latter being connected to a common grounded point, the shield of the cabinet. This arrangement reduces the effective tension between any point and the electrical cabinet. Thus the insulation costs are lowered and the safety is improved. This is shown in figure 6.4.

The transformer core must be able to handle high levels of electromagnetic induction, so they are made from grain-oriented sheets. The transformer is completely immersed in a special transformer oil, which has a high insulating power and also allows for good thermal conduction. It is therefore used in the dissipation of the heat produced by the high powers present. In some transformers sulfur hexafluoride gas is used for insulation because it does not break down over time and is lighter than the oil.

Together with the high voltage transformer is installed a transformer whose secondary side feeds the filament of the x-ray tubes. The primary voltage of this transformer comes from the generator and determines the current (mA) which will flow through the tube.

The rectifier system is located inside the cabinet, usually connected by a bridge of special high voltage semiconductor diodes (first-generation devices used valves as rectifiers). In addition it includes a system of switches, used to direct the high voltage

Technical Fundamentals of Radiology and CT

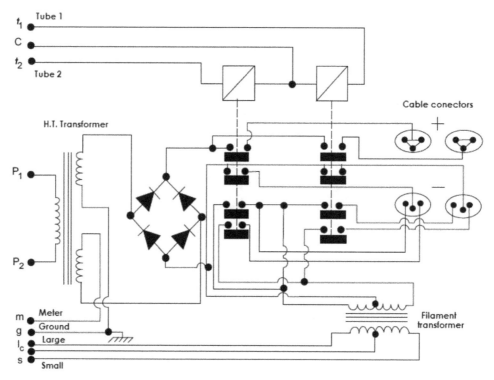

Figure 6.5. A high voltage transformer circuit.

to one or more x-ray tubes, and other switches that change the voltage from one filament to the other. This circuit is shown in figure 6.5.

The female terminals that receive the high voltage cables are located on the outer surface of the cabinet. These terminals are unique and are manufactured with materials of high dielectric strength, and they fit exactly into the male terminals of the high tension cables, which are inserted after conditioning them with special silicone. One terminal carries the positive voltage to the anode and the other carries the negative voltage to the cathode of the tube with a bifilar filament voltage supply.

In the same cabinet are installed the strip connecting cables coming into the high voltage transformer system from the generator: the cables for primary high voltage, and the cables that control the switching of tubes and the switching of filaments in both tubes (large, small, common). The configuration described is the most common, although some manufacturers incorporate other functions and devices in the cabinet, such as the remote fluoroscopic control voltage.

6.9.1 The transformation ratio

From the electrical standpoint, the transformer performs conversion from a low voltage to a higher level or vice versa. In some cases transformers that do not change the relationship of the voltages or out-windings are only used as separators. In most cases, the high voltage transformer is only used as a voltage elevator, that is, the output is much higher than the input voltage.

The transformation ratio gives us, in practical terms, the output voltage ranging from 40 000 V (40 kV) to 150 000 V (150 kV) from the input voltages to the autotransformer, in which they are between 180 V and 350 V. The transformation ratio is mathematically simple and is expressed in terms of input and output voltages to the number of turns of the primary and secondary windings. The relevant equation is as follows:

$$\frac{V_1}{V_2} = \frac{N_1}{N_2},$$

V_1 and V_2 being the input and output voltages, respectively, and N_1 and N_2 the number of turns of the primary and secondary windings, respectively. From the above equation it can be seen that to have a high output voltage there should be a lot of turns in the secondary winding, which reiterates the above mentioned necessity of carefully isolation.

6.10 Rectification and power

Everything related to the conversion of the alternating voltage, as a continuous voltage applied to the x-ray tube, is known as rectification. This concept involves obtaining a voltage which varies only in one direction, the alternating voltage being a voltage that varies in both directions, positive and negative. If the alternating voltage is applied to the tube for a second cycle, the anode would be positive and the next cycle would be negative. This would result in the impact of accelerated electrons on the anode and subsequently a possible emission of electrons torn by the high field from the anode and their impact on the cathode, causing it to deteriorate. As this situation is unsustainable, it is necessary to only have electrons flow in one direction, from the cathode to the anode. Fortunately the physical constitution of the tube allows only the latter possibility, so the tube itself becomes a rectifier, which is why in small devices the tube itself performs the rectification.

6.10.1 Self-rectification

Self-rectified systems are defined as x-ray systems that do not use rectifiers. The power is not fully used, because during half the cycle the tube has reversed polarity and does not produce rays. Therefore, self-rectifiers do not have applications in medium to high power devices. There is also the disadvantage that they cannot implement all the high voltage permitted by the tube. This is explained by the fact that during conduction a high voltage is applied between the electrodes, but when there is no conduction that voltage is in a vacuum. That is, the voltage is not decreased, so it has a real value higher than the previous one, raising the risk of destruction by internal discharge in the tube. This requires the tube to work at a lower real value of nominal kilovolts; for example, a specified maximum voltage tube of 125 kV would have to work at real value not exceeding 100 kV [10].

Another drawback of this system is the fact that the pulsating rectified current flows through the loop comprising the secondary winding of the transformer,

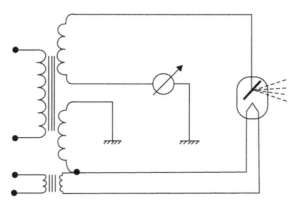

Figure 6.6. A self-rectifying x-ray tube circuit.

generating a component of continuous voltage which saturates the core. This reduces the conversion efficiency which necessitates the use of oversized transformers. Figure 6.6 shows the circuit of a single self-rectifying x-ray tube.

6.10.2 Half-wave rectification

Half-wave rectification circuits are used only in low power devices. The rectifier is a device that only allows driving in one direction, so that upon inputting an alternating voltage a pulse voltage is obtained. The first rectifiers used for x-rays were called Kenotrons or gas rectifiers which have now been replaced by the use of solid-state rectifier diodes made of silicon or selenium. Their comparative advantages are such that they have completely eliminated the use of other forms of rectification.

Solid-state rectifiers are widely used today. Selenium rectifiers were initially used, but have the problem of causing a high internal voltage drop. Modern devices use only silicon rectifiers. It should be noted that the rectifiers used in radiology have a unique elongated cylindrical shape with the connectors at the ends, and obviously must have the property of being able to withstand high reverse voltages.

In practical circuits of half-wave rectification two diodes are used in series with the ends of the transformer. This enables overcoming some of the problems of self-rectification systems in the x-ray tube. For example, the maximum rated voltage can now be applied to the tube and the risk of generating anode electrons is avoided. However, the problem of having to apply a double current to achieve the desired dose persists, this is explained by the fact that driving occurs for only a half cycle of the ac signal. Figure 6.7 shows the circuit of a half-wave rectifier with two diodes.

It is clear that there will be higher performance if the rectified voltage is applied to the tube throughout the electrical circulation cycle, therefore specific circuits are necessary to obtain full-wave rectification.

6.10.3 Full-wave rectification

Full-wave rectification can be obtained by means of a Graetz bridge system, which will always have a pulsed wave output during the whole cycle. This system is widely

Technical Fundamentals of Radiology and CT

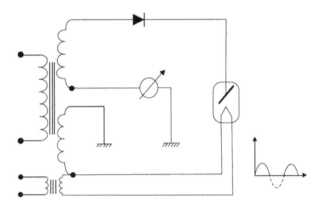

Figure 6.7. A half-wave rectification circuit.

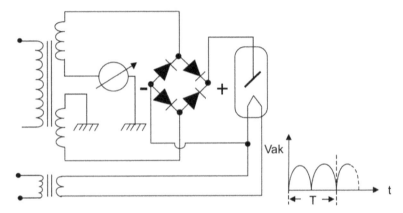

Figure 6.8. A full-wave rectification circuit.

used in conventional electronic rectifiers and is also applied successfully in high voltage rectification systems (see figure 6.8). With this circuit some significant advantages can be achieved. The x-ray tube does not have to withstand any reverse voltage, since it only receives a pulsed voltage with a positive charge always applied to the anode. It has superior performance in terms of the use of the energy contained in a complete cycle, since the two adjacent half-waves are at a higher level of energy than that obtained by the half-wave rectifier system. Moreover, with a higher average applied voltage, the dose is increased and better performance is obtained with a lower tube current.

However, this system still has some drawbacks due to the fact that a dc voltage is not applied to the tube. The fluctuation in half-sine shape implies a waste of potential energy in the region between voltage peaks, which has the drawback of influencing the minimum duration of the radiation. It follows that the ideal waveform with respect to time and radiation dose is a continuous wave, in which the maximum voltage is set to zero time and the wave always has uniform tension throughout the complete cycle.

6-11

The theoretical solution to this problem is achieving perfect multiphase rectification or applying a high dc voltage. The latter solution is unattainable through ac mains and electronic filtering, as used in low voltage circuits, so the first solution is the most practically applicable. Another original and theoretically valid solution is the use of frequencies higher than the network input, so that the correction immediately obtains a pulsed wave [11] with minimum ripple. The latter is technologically complex and requires the use of saturable core transformers and dc–ac converters. This increases the complexity and decreases the reliability of the system.

The most commonly used system before the invention of high frequency systems (known as multipulse) was polyphase rectification, a solution that improves the performance through sequenced rectifiers. There are systems with six alternating phases and six rectifiers, six alternating phases and twelve rectifiers, and twelve alternating phases with twelve rectifiers.

6.10.4 Three-phase rectifiers

Having an alternating fixed frequency signal in the network limits the possibility of increasing the ripple of the rectified wave; theoretically the wave ripple cannot be improved if additional filtering does not occur, which is not possible as the capacitors require support by a tension value greater than the maximum voltage applied to the tube, technically an almost unattainable aim [12]. So another solution is applied to the load, in this case the x-ray tube, a series of pulses out-of-phase so that the path of descent of the peak to the next pulse is smaller than in the sequence of the full wave. A graphical interpretation of events helps in understanding the out-of-phase process, which is caused by the action of the secondary windings of a three-phase transformer that is connected to a star, so that the angular relationship between them is 180°. That is, the pulse sequence is such that the closeness between the peaks for each phase pulse is greater. In short, while in a system of one-phase full-wave rectification there are two peaks and two levels of zero in a complete cycle, in a three-phase system there are six peaks and six minimum differences of zero per cycle.

6.10.5 A three-phase system with six pulses and six rectifiers

A system of this type uses a primary input of three-phase in a delta connection, with three secondary windings in star-connection, with the center point of the star connected to ground; each winding end is connected to two rectifier diodes in parallel (see figure 6.9). Each cable of the three-phase secondary winding is connected to the cathode of one diode and simultaneously to the anode of another diode. Thus the resulting wave is a sequence of six pulses in one cycle. The ripple of this system is superior to that of a one-phase full-wave system, but in practice the theoretical value obtained deteriorates with the load to which the circuit is subjected.

An assembly that improves the above-described is obtained by means of a circuit using the same type of primary delta connection, and a pair of separated star windings on the secondary side, see figure 6.10. This arrangement provides a path in series for the two stars windings near the x-ray tube, so that, by having the

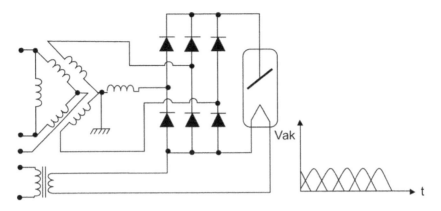

Figure 6.9. A three-phase, six-pulse and six-rectifier circuit.

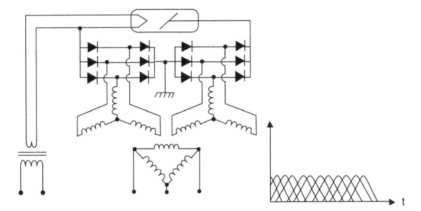

Figure 6.10. A three-phase, six-pulse, twelve rectifier circuit.

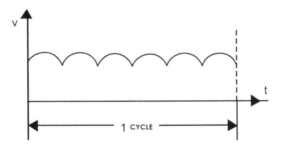

Figure 6.11. The ripple shape of the rectified wave.

point of both systems connected to ground, the two halves are applied to the tube adding the total voltage, thereby sharing the total load between each star. This assembly is expensive, but as it allows the circuit to obtain the advantages of symmetrical and balanced distribution of the load by the ripple at full conduction, it is better than the previously described circuits, as shown in figure 6.11.

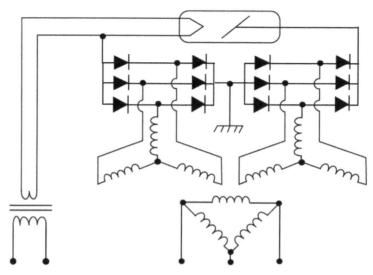

Figure 6.12. A three-phase, twelve-pulse and twelve-rectifier circuit.

6.10.6 A three-phase system with twelve pulses and twelve rectifiers

The way to obtain higher rectification efficiency is to increase the number of pulses per cycle, so that the resultant wave has the largest possible energy content with a smaller difference between the peak and minimum. The practical way to achieve this is by producing a correction of twelve pulses per cycle, which is possible if we phase out 30° in the outputs of the secondary windings. The way to achieve this is to connect one secondary in a delta configuration and the other in a star configuration. The resulting waveform is the best of all those studied and so the ripple factor is minimized at full load (see figure 6.12).

In summary, the possible ways to obtain rectification are:
- Self-rectification.
- Half-wave rectification with a double diode.
- Full-wave rectification with four diodes.
- Three-phase rectification with six pulses and six diodes.
- Three-phase rectification with six pulses and twelve diodes.
- Three-phase rectification with twelve pulses and twelve diodes.

The most modern system used to obtain high voltage is based on the generation of a different frequency to that of the network, in the range of 20–50 kHz, thereby better results and better efficiency are obtained. This system will be studied in chapter 12.

6.11 High voltage cables

Carrying the high voltage from the transformer to the tube requires solving the problem of how to handle the high electric tension. Obviously the tube cannot be placed at the same point as the transformer, there must be the possibility to handle the tube in proximity to the patient, elevate it, tilt it to different angles [13], etc. Therefore special cables are required to carry the voltage, which can withstand the high voltages to be applied to the tube. Moreover, the cable connected to the tube on the cathode side must also carry the power supply to the filament.

All high voltage cables must have adequate insulation of high dielectric strength, mechanical protection against breakage or tensile strains and the flexibility to allow manipulation of the tube. This makes the construction of these cables a specialized electromechanical task, especially in relation to the high electrical insulation required (see figure 6.13).

All high voltage cables have standardized terminals at both ends, one to be connected to the female terminals of the high voltage transformer and another to be connected to the female terminals located in the tube housing. The coupling must be perfect, including silicone gel for isolation and adjusted by means of threaded rings that are tightened at both ends. In the practice of radiology some cases of cables damaged through misuse are known, so careful management is recommended, particularly when the column moves with the tube, since most the failures are caused by mechanical damage and the deterioration of isolation.

High voltage cables are manufactured with the following options according to its terminals (see figures 6.14 and 6.15):
 – GE TYPE.
 – FED STD II.
 – SP-120, SP-140.
 – XRD.

The lengths most used are 1.5, 3, 4.5, 6, 7.5, 9, 10.5, 12, 14, 15, 17 and 18 meters.
They can also be manufactured with a length specified by the user. The diameters used are: 2, 2.2 and 2.5 centimeters. The cable insulation is defined with respect to the ground and not in relation to the voltage to be carried by the tube, its values are between 75 kVp and 120 kVp.

6.12 The radiographic tube

A complete system, of course, includes one or more x-ray tubes. It is common to find only one tube in a simple installation, called a radiographic system, since its

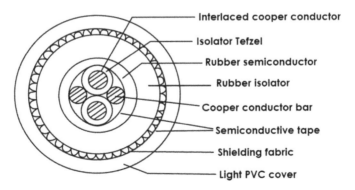

Figure 6.13. Internal construction of a high voltage cable.

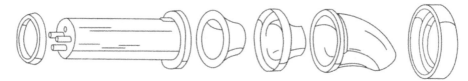

STANDARD TYPE II TERMINAL

Figure 6.14. Terminals of a high voltage cable and its components.

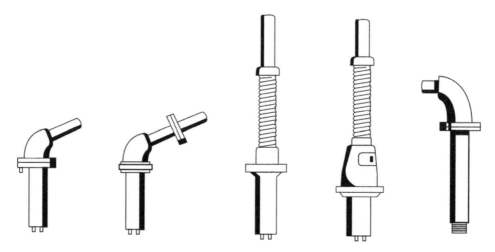

Figure 6.15. Different types of terminals for high voltage cables.

sole function is to produce radiographs. This is different from a fluoroscopy tube. Although it also generates x-rays, its name arises from its specific application to visualize by fluoroscopic radiation the region which is to be subsequently radiographed.

We will not delve further into the tubes, which are already described above, but we emphasize the fact that an x-ray tube must be installed in a way that allows one to obtain films or images from a patient lying on a table or standing against a cassette hanger on the wall, and also the use of any other device (which generally defines the name of the system), such as the previously described surgical C-arm, mammography, R/F, tomography, etc. All are defined by the specific function they perform and where the tube is in relation to the patient, and other factors such as the sequence of radiographic shots.

Some systems require the installation of two tubes, one for each level of study, as in some cardiovascular devices. Others usually carry a 'fluoroscopic' tube [14] under the table and a 'radiographic' tube on a mobile stand (as shown in figures 6.16 and 6.17). There are also facilities that use three tubes with the same generator, although this is less common.

Technical Fundamentals of Radiology and CT

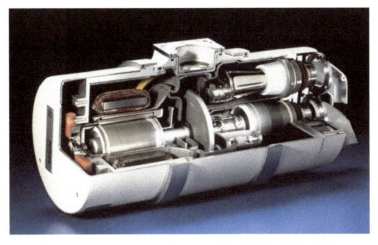

Figure 6.16. An x-ray tube. Courtesy of Koninklijke Philips N. V.

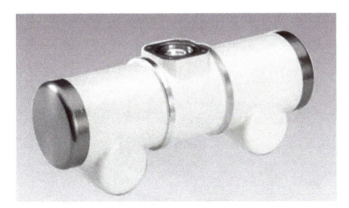

Figure 6.17. A fluoroscopic tube. Courtesy of Siemens.

6.13 Electromechanical accessories

Radiation should be applied to patients who are positioned comfortably and appropriately for the study being performed. This is possible if there are other devices that complement the function of the generator and tube. The idea is to have a good installation to provide better working conditions and guarantee the best results, since most radiological studies require a specific set of conditions to be met. Among these accessories are the radiographic table, the stand column that supports and moves tubes throughout the installation, the cassette hanger or Bucky anti-scatter system for chest radiographs, the rails for ceiling tube holders or to support TV systems, the carriages for monitors and mechanical supports for positioning trauma patients. Of all these devices, the most frequently used are radiographic tables. Other important components are specialized contrast injectors with electronic control, electromechanical systems working as film changers with a high work sequence and other advanced systems for further radiological processing, such as digital subtraction angiography (DSA) devices, systems for video recording of images, cine-radiographic projectors, film developers, and so on.

6.14 Radiographic tables

The tables used in radiology can be of different types, from simple and light tables similar to stretchers, to those endowed with great technical sophistication. The latter can, for example, position the patient in many ways [15], make serial radiographs, allow subdivision of films and contain TV systems, and generally allow the widest variety of procedures used in contemporary radiology. There are also simple tilting tables that are mainly used in emergency rooms.

The simplest table is one that supports the patient only horizontally, without the possibility of moving in any direction, and is only applicable for moving the tube over the patient in the region to be radiographed (figures 6.18 and 6.19).

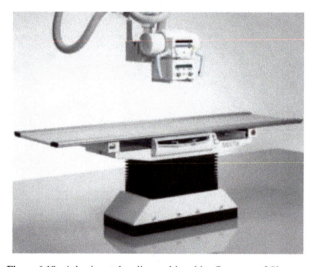

Figure 6.18. A horizontal radiographic table. Courtesy of Siemens.

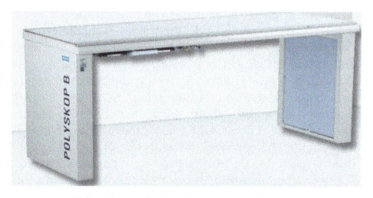

Figure 6.19. A simple table. Courtesy of Siemens.

Among the features of simple horizontal radiographic tables, are the following:
- Table top dimensions of the order of 70 cm × 200 cm (28 inches × 80 inches).
- A distance between the table top and the film of the order of 2 to 2.5 cm (or 7/8 to 1 inch).
- A bottom bracket for anti-scatter (Bucky) and a maximum dimensions tray plate holder cassette (the radiographic chassis).
- Patient immobilization supports.
- Some tables have a top cover with movement in the longitudinal direction and optionally in the lateral direction.
- An electromagnetic brake using a pedal or manual action to activate or block the longitudinal and lateral movements.
- The surface height of these tables is about 75 cm (30 inches) and can be adjusted to a certain extent during installation.
- The filtering effect of radiation on the table is equivalent to no more than 1 mm of aluminum.

Simple tables with these features are used for general examinations and simple routine orthopedic examination.

The more complex tables have the following classification:
1. Simple tilting tables.
2. Fluoroscopic tilting tables.
3. Remotely controlled tables.
4. Tomographic tables.
5. Tables for special studies (angiography, urology, etc).

6.14.1 Simple tilting tables

These tables are unique in that they tilt on their axis, allowing studies with the patient positioned horizontally, vertically, or tilted with his/her head downward in the so-called Trendelenburg position, with a limit of 15° below the horizontal line. These tables have an electrical circuit that allows the tilting movement to be motorized and are properly balanced to immobilize the table in the last position if power failure should occur, with security systems to stop the movement when the limits of each position (horizontal, vertical, Trendelenburg) are achieved. Some simple tilting tables also have a top board that is movable in the longitudinal and lateral directions using a motor located somewhere on the base.

In summary, the features of simple tilting tables are:
- Motorized tilting of 90°–15°.
- An optionally fixed or mobile board with a range of approximately 60 cm (24 inches).
- An anti-scatter (Bucky) grid in an electric counterbalanced position.
- A tray for various dimensions of cassette films.
- A top board made of a material that is translucent to x-rays.
- Removable feet and removable handles for support.
- Tilt controls with easy access.

6-19

- Safety switches to stop the motion on reaching the limits.
- Some have a built-in retractable step to access to the patient.
- Lead weights or springs to maintain the table in any position with or without power.
- Compression clamping fixtures for the patient, such as chest compression bands, head fasteners, infant immobilizers, etc.

6.14.2 Fluoroscopic tilting tables

This is currently the most widely used table in routine radiological work. It incorporates a special feature, the device used for subdivisions of radiographic films. This table accessory is also known as the spot film device and is described in detail in section 7.4.

This type of table does not differ significantly from the simple one. It also has tilt and shift of the cover board, a counterbalanced Bucky, sensors for safety limits and all the characteristics that were defined for simple tilt tables. Fluoroscopic tables also have an automatic cut-off limit of the tilt on reaching the horizontal position from any angle lower or higher than zero. This allows the operator to obtain an automatic zero positioning angle without having to constantly control the angle indicator, thus speeding up their work.

These tables have a fluoroscopic x-ray tube located under the table [16], which is integrally connected to the spot film device, such that they move together laterally and longitudinally. The purpose of such an arrangement is to mobilize both components so as to locate and select the region studied by the operator, keeping the patient between the x-ray tube and the film contained in the spot film device.

The mounting of the spot film on the table requires counterweights for easy mobilization in all directions, that is, up and down and in the longitudinal and lateral directions, as required. Once the region of interest is located, the spot film should be immobilize in the chosen position by the electromagnetic brakes. These tables include a circuit that immediately activates certain brakes when the center position with respect to the table is reached. The system can automatically locate the position of the spot film allowing better utilization of the film into several divisions, as in panoramic shots.

Fluoroscopic tables allow the use of the x-ray tube located under the table for screen or TV displays [17] and recording the body parts to be documented on radiographic film, hence the tube is used for dual functions in both fluoroscopic and radiographic modes. This requires specific circuits in the spot film device that commute the tube function at the time of making the radiographic shot.

The image intensifier system for TV images (which is switchable with a video camera and a fixed photo camera with a film of 100 mm) can be installed in the spot film device. In the design of spot film devices, consideration should be given to the increased weight, and balance should be obtained for the accessories responsible for the weight increase. The control of the table must be multi-functional, combining the controls for tilting the table and the spot film device.

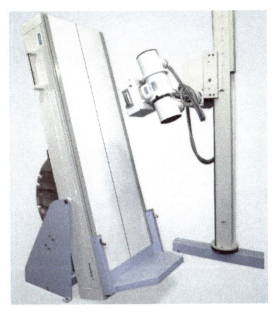

Figure 6.20. A simple tilting table. Courtesy of Siemens.

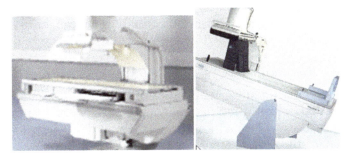

Figure 6.21. A fluoroscopic tilt table. Courtesy of Siemens.

Thus the operator can use the spot film for all functions and control the movements of the table, and the opening or closing of collimator plates connected to the tube, without moving away from the device. Fluoroscopic tables have a motor circuit which helps in the longitudinal displacement of the spot film at one or more speeds. This is particularly useful when the table is used in a vertical position (see figure 6.20).

Fluoroscopic tables have the great disadvantage of the mechanical complexity of the subdivision of films and the tilting system. These features entail various problems for maintenance, due to the constant contact and rubbing of mechanical parts, such as sheets for restriction, transport systems, movements of the film holder and gears, and other systems [18]. Modern devices are tending toward the

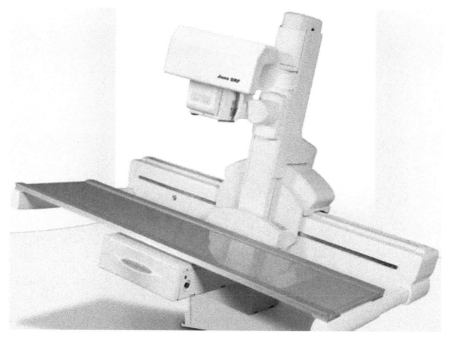

Figure 6.22. A remotely controlled tilting table. Courtesy of Siemens.

digital manipulation of different formats instead of the mechanical functions used in this type of table, as with the R/F conventional table shown in figure 6.21.

6.14.3 Remotely controlled tables

One of the most significant advances in terms of patient manipulation has been the arrival of remotely controlled tables (see figure 6.22). By their nature these tables allow all kinds of tests to be performed under conditions of greater freedom and radiation safety for the personnel who are permanently working in, and therefore may be subjected to, a harmful radiogenic load.

In addition to remote control of the table [19], the most notable difference between these tables and those described above is the fact that the tube is placed over the patient and not under the table; this feature was explained in section 4.4.3. Among the advantages of remote controlled tables is the ability to move the image intensifier [20] so that the examination can be performed from the patient's feet to their head without moving him/her. Another significant advantage is the possibility to take tomographic images and perform studies using films changers. Tables of this type have a special ultrafast spot film system and an automatic light collimator with centering at several depths. A column tube stand that moves longitudinally is attached to the table and is used for tomographic studies or to achieve any angle in zonographic images (tomographic studies in a specific area). One type of remotely controlled table also has a compression device which is operated by remote control. This informs the operator of the patient's reactions through feedback and helps to move the contrast liquid in the stomach. Despite the ability to remotely control the table, the system must have an additional control located in the table itself. The range of remote control is large and allows all kinds of possibilities, making this type of table a powerful tool for radiological studies.

Among the main control functions of remotely controlled tables are:

- The controls and display for the table.
- A control panel with a push button for fluoroscopy connection and disconnection.
- Moving the image intensifier.
- Variation of the focal length.
- Tilting the table.
- Oblique incidence of radiation.
- Position selector controls.
- A schedule of formats.
- The availability of digital displays of radiographs.
- Cassette input and output.
- Automatic collimation with focused light.
- Adjusting the angle of a tomography slice.
- Digital display of the cutting plane.
- A selector for the cutting plane.
- A patient compressor.
- A TV camera and still camera.
- Brightness and contrast control.
- Manual and/or automatic dose control.
- Image inversion.
- A field selector.
- Time selection and photographic cadence.
- An exposure and remaining films counter.

6.15 Tomography

Even when full systems, such as the R/F radiographic tables described above, enable linear tomographic studies using an accessory that longitudinally attaches to the tube and film cassette, there are devices that have special tomographic functions in order to perform specific and complex zonographic studies, with any angle, depth, or location of the tomographic plane. These accessories allow the realization of linear, circular and elliptical scans at different speeds. Before describing the function of these tables it is essential to understand the fundamental concept of tomography; this is also necessary for understanding CT scan technology, which is currently the most important diagnostic tool in radiology.

Tomography arises from the way in which radiographic images are presented on a film. Overlapping planes and x-ray structures can be confused such that the plane to be observed appears along with other planes that are not useful. This radiological practice is overcome by the knowledge of diagnostic patterns that the radiologist has, so he/she can assess the necessary plane in an image while disregarding the presence of other planes. However, in many cases certain delicate structures, such as the fine bones of the ear, some intracranial cavities and parts of the digestive system,

Technical Fundamentals of Radiology and CT

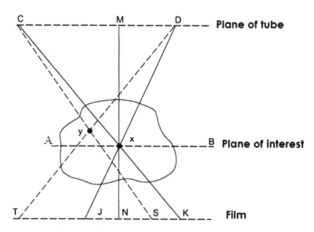

Figure 6.23. The linear tomography principle.

and in general any specific structure which needs to be displayed clearly, requires an image without the effects caused by the presence of other planes. The solution to obtain a sharp image plane is to blur all the planes that are not of interest, keeping only the necessary structures of the body in focus. This is accomplished by moving the tube while it produces radiation, together with the film which moves in the opposite direction.

While in conventional imaging the goal is to prevent movement of the tube and the film, in tomography, movement is produced deliberately to reduce the definition of all structures below and above the level of examination. The clarity of the desired plane is achieved by the fact that a geometric center of rotation remains where the x-rays always pass without horizontal scrolling. That is, this geometric center appears as if it were a pivotal axis, which means that the image obtained in the desired plane appears as if the tube and film have not been moved. Obviously, the results are not perfect in practice, as the useless planes next to the plane of interest always have some degree of influence on the film. However, the results are sufficiently good to allow diagnoses.

Analysis of the graph in figure 6.23 allows a better understanding of the principle of linear tomography. The plane to study located in the patient is defined as the length A–B, and we assume that the tube and the film holder, located at the ends of the line M–N, move as one, and may occupy the possible positions between C–D and J–K. If the rotation has axis at point X (the center of rotation or the fulcrum), there will always be x-rays passing through it, whatever the position of the tube and the film. Then the projection of the image will only be clear at the points that are in the plane parallel to the film in accordance with point X. The geometric explanation is as follows: for all points of the plane at the height of the fulcrum, there is a relation of similarity between the triangle formed by the length between the tube and the perpendicular plane (C–X), the line of travel of the tube to the fulcrum (M–X) and the semi-displacement of the tube (C–M), with the triangle formed by the distance between the fulcrum and film (X–K), the perpendicular to the plane of the film from the fulcrum (X–N) and the semi-travel of the film (N–K). The triangles formed by MXD and XNK also maintain similarity. This applies to all points of the A–B plane, which projects its image over the plate in the same way for any position of the tube and the film. This is not the case for points located outside the plane, such as point Y which at the initial position of the tube casts its shadow at point S, and in the end position casts its shadow at point T. As can be seen, the greater distance between J and T will result in greater blurring for the image corresponding to point Y. The plane we are interested in can be selected through the coincidence of the plane with the fulcrum, which is physically accessible using the mobilization bar of the tube. Such a coincidence of the plane can be obtained through using a moving table with the patient on it.

As explained above, there is a degree of thickness which is reflected in the film, i.e. not only does the level of interest appear clearly, but also the neighboring planes. In practice the goal is to reduce this thickness greatly by moving the tube and the film holder; this is explained by the fact that the angle that has as its sides the lines between the tube in its extreme and fulcrum positions, determines the thickness that comes out on the film, the larger the angle is, the lower the thickness. This can be seen in figure 6.24 where angle α determines a clear region between MNOP and angle β determines a larger clear region between M'N'O'P'. Large angle tomography is called planigraphy and other types of tomography that use a small angle (on the order of 5°) are known as zonography [21].

The realization of tomography involves taking into account some important aspects:
- A higher dose than in conventional x-rays should be applied, which is justified by the fact that the radiation must traverse a greater thickness at certain tube positions, and the focus–film distance increases when the tube is separated from the center of rotation.
- Planigraphic radiation times are higher than those used in conventional radiography, because the duration of the system's motion is much higher than that of the conventional longest shot.

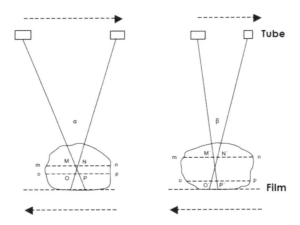

Figure 6.24. Tomographic angle and sharpness.

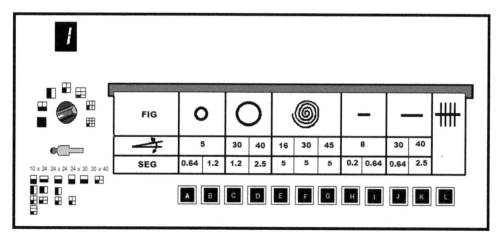

Figure 6.25. A tomography system. Courtesy of Siemens.

- The system requires that the correct parallel is always maintained between the film holder and the tube.
- The patient must lie still for the duration of the scan.

6.15.1 Tomographic systems

The linear scan described above is not the only way to perform tomography, as there are other ways to cause the desired blurring of the planes that are not of interest, and other forms of tomographic studies with complex movements of the whole tube–film system exist, which can be selected in the control panel, similar to that shown in figure 6.25. These movements can be:
- Linear.
- Arc.
- Circular.
- Spiral.
- Lace.
- Ellipse.
- Helical.

Figure 6.26, depicts a basic tomography system showing the table, the motor drive system, the tomograph bar, the turret and control cabinet.

6.15.2 The motor drive system

The motor drive system is the device responsible for producing the tomographic displacement, by means of a motor that transmits movement to a column tube or a ceiling support bracket. The rotation ratio is designed to move the tube from one end to another of the table over the patient, keeping the given focal length [22]. A linear scan produces radiation during the forward movement and the return to

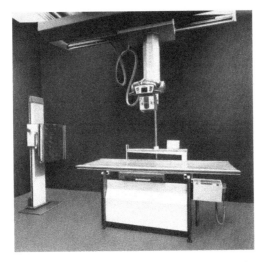

Figure 6.26. A basic tomography system. Courtesy of Siemens.

the initial position does not involve radiation. All types of motors should have a system without mechanical tolerances based on a chain drive and they should not have an articulated arm for rotation. The movement should be smooth and without vibration so it must be mounted on ball bearings.

6.15.3 The tomograph bar

The tomograph bar is fitted between the tube holder and the support column containing the anti-scatter film holder. Its function is to transmit the longitudinal movement to the film in solidarity with the tube when it moves in the opposite direction. This addition converts a conventional table into a tomographic table, so most equipment manufacturers include the possibility to make this conversion in their tables. Obviously, when a system is required that allows studies to be conducted at different depths and speeds, and with different forms of movement and various divisions in the film, a specialized device, or multitomograph, is required, as with the system shown in figure 6.27.

6.15.4 Turret

The turret is the component intended to define the center of rotation of the bar and adjust the height of the patient body corresponding to the plane to be x-rayed. This turret is mounted on a conventional table or is fixed in specialized tomographs.

6.15.5 Control cabinet

The control cabinet is designed to contain the circuitry to select the travel speed, the type of scan and also choose whether or not to apply the tomographic motion to table. It is usually mounted on a wall or on any side of the table where it can be operated easily.

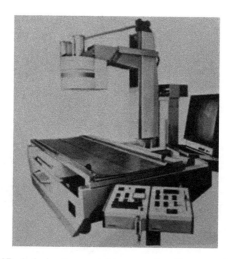

Figure 6.27. A device for special tomography. Courtesy of Siemens.

6.15.6 Multidirectional tomograph

This specialized tomograph has a set of specific features, including:
- The possibility of more than ten paths.
- Motorized height adjustment in values millimeter by millimeter.
- Optical display of the cutting height via a projection beam on the patient.
- A wide range of adjustable tomographic heights.
- Angle control.
- Control of movement times.
- Automated selection of film sizes and subdivisions.
- Automatic collimation.
- Scan type selections.
- A sliding patient table (motorized or manual).
- Optional automatic control dosage.

Some tomography systems have the ability to make longitudinal, lateral and oblique projections using a C-arm system and table on a pivotal point, keeping the iso-center level throughout the C-arm rotation.

References

[1] General Electric Medical Systems 1983 X-ray generators *Training Course*
[2] General Electric Medical Systems 1998 MST 1050 X-ray unit *Service Manual* SM A0655
[3] General Electric Medical Systems 1998 DXD 325 X ray *Service Manual* SM A0653A
[4] Pickel G 1969 La automatización en la radio técnica el TRIOMAT *Rev. SRW* **3** 16–22
[5] Biehl H and Zier W 1973 Progresos en los generadores de radiodiagnóstico *Med. Technik* **4** 116–28
[6] Centro Nacional de Información en Ciencias Médicas 1979 Qué es un aparato de rayos X tipo condensador *Temas de Electrónica* (Havana: Centro Nacional de Información en Ciencias Médicas)

[7] Pickel G 1970 El Tridoros 5, un nuevo tipo de aparato trifásico para el diagnóstico *Rev. SRW* **1** 5–16

[8] Friedel R and Geldner E 1986 Características de calidad de los modernos emisores de rayos X reflejadas en la normalización *Electromédica* **3** 76–80

[9] Billege I 1969 The latest x-ray equipment of Medicor works *Medicor News* **1** 1–14

[10] General Electric Medical Systems 1986 Mobile '200' type 2 x-ray unit *Service Engineering Handbook*

[11] Universal X-Ray Inc. 1986 How to assemble the Easymatic 125, 300 and 325 mobile x-ray unit Service *Manual* #083074

[12] Zamora D 2013 Basics of x-ray and mammography systems University of Washington School of Medicine Course http://courses.washington.edu/radxphys/

[13] Claumount Assemblies 1987 Small diameter x-ray cable assemblies Spec No. C-1311769 B

[14] Wolter 1977 Loadix, sistema para el control térmico de emisores de rayos X *Electromedica* **2** 73–6

[15] General Electric Medical Systems 1996 RT *table Product Data* B 7010

[16] General Electric Spain 1987 Genematic, mesa para radiodiagnóstico *Catalog* A-401

[17] Gayler B W and Donner M W 1972 El orbiskop, un nuevo equipo de fluoroscopia *Electromédica* **1** 4–13

[18] General Electric Medical systems 1987 Fluoricon compact, Monitrol 15 standard R & F systems *Catalog* **50001R**

[19] Schwarz G and Schmidt E 1979 Course of the examination and result of ERCP carried out on a remote controlled x-ray unit *Electromedica* **4** 161–4

[20] General Electric Medical Systems 1997 Telegem 11 mesa basculante telemandada *Product Data* **1330** 3132

[21] Marx E 1974 La zonografía en el diagnóstico de las vías urinarias *Electromédica* **4** 101–9

[22] Gebauer A 1979 The x-ray planigraphic examination of the abdomen *Electromédica* **3** 105–8

IOP Publishing

Technical Fundamentals of Radiology and CT

Guillermo Avendaño Cervantes

Chapter 7

Electromechanical accessories

This chapter examines some electromechanical accessories of great importance that are used in radiology to complement the devices described in previous chapters.

7.1 The wall cassette holder with an anti-scatter grid

This wall cassette holder is used for obtaining radiographs with the patient standing or sitting (see figure 7.1). In some cases this device is used for tests ranging from the lower extremities to the skull, but the most common use is to obtain chest x-rays.

The basic vertical support comprises a column which is fixed to the floor and wall with a vertically sliding plate holder approximately 100 cm in length. The cassette plate can be installed effortlessly directly or through a side slot on the cassette holder from the front. In some cases the system has a Bucky grid, which can move forward in a gradual trajectory of 0–20° to carry out specific techniques and tilt to the horizontal position for studies of the extremities. Both the full anti-scatter grid as well as the single tray cassette holder have a system of counterweights which balance the system and move it effortlessly, and some devices also have mechanical or electromagnetic brake positioning [1].

This device has grooved brackets on both sides in order to allow installation of standardized accessories. Normally, the brackets allow the addition of different types of anti-scatter grids and the possibility of installing an automatic dose exposimeter [2].

7.2 Column tube stand

The purpose of a column tube stand is apparent from its name. It can be used to position or move the x-ray tube to the patient if on a table, or position the tube towards a wall holder.

doi:10.1088/978-0-7503-1212-7ch7   7-1   © IOP Publishing Ltd 2016

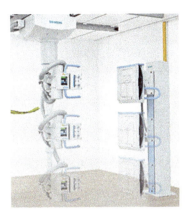

Figure 7.1. A wall cassette holder with counterbalanced Bucky supports. Courtesy of Siemens.

The most important features of these columns are:
- The possibility of rotating the tube with respect to the two axes, vertical and horizontal.
- A horizontal arm with telescoping displacement which can be locked every 90° in each rotation of the shaft column.
- A numerical display of all movable distances.
- A counterweight system for the movement through weights or a spring system.
- Electromagnetic braking and safety devices to protect against cable breakage through traction.
- The possibility of supporting the column on rails on the floor and a sliding wall or ceiling [3], in the first case it is called a wall–floor column and in the second a floor–ceiling column.
- Suitable support and safety clamps for the tube.
- Clamps for the different wires present (high voltage, brake supply for light collimator, etc) so that the wires do not tangle and to prevent any possibility of destroying them through the movement of the column.
- These columns usually have an upper extension of the height to adjust the column to the ceiling height of the location where it is to be installed.

Column tube stands have a head with a command handle in which are located the brake switch which stops the tube in any of the selected positions, a goniometer indicating the inclination of the tube relative to the table and some type of visual indication to monitor column performance. In some models the head includes light control of the collimator. Some systems provide visual indication when the displacement reaches the exact standardized distances for x-rays on the table or on the anti-scatter device (100 cm or 183 cm). In figure 7.2 a classic column tube stand is displayed.

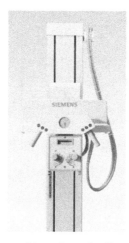

Figure 7.2. A stand column with a tube and collimator. Courtesy of Siemens.

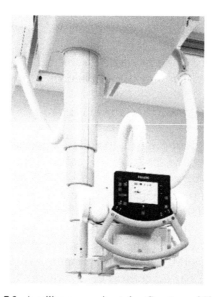

Figure 7.3. A ceiling suspension tube. Courtesy of Siemens.

7.3 Ceiling suspensions

In many facilities it is of interest to be able to move the tube in the entire available space for the purpose of performing any kind of study at the ends of a table or against various wall holders. For this purpose a suspension system is installed which allows full mobilization of a tube (see figure 7.3). The positioning is performed manually on the tube itself through some clamps connected to the tube support or

Technical Fundamentals of Radiology and CT

the end of the collimator. These are very close to the controls for the brakes, allowing easy manipulation.

All ceiling support systems should have:
- Wide longitudinal and transverse local coverage.
- A telescopic column with a displacement of approximately 150 cm.
- A vibration-free column, this is achieved using a polygonal telescopic system with self-aligning bearings.
- A customizable universal support for any kind of ceiling, with an L or H profile.
- An inertial break counterbalance system or traction cables for safety.
- Positioning and electromagnetic brakes.
- Tube clamps and/or a removable image intensifier system.
- A system connecting the rails on the ceiling [4], which can be external or internal. In the first case there is a stationary rail which enables movement of the bearing frame, which is at the same level as the structure. An internally bearing system also has a stationary rail, but the frame is on the outside of the stationary rail. Both systems are chosen according to local specifications and customer needs. Figures 7.4 and 7.5 show the two types of ceiling support.

7.4 The spot film device

We have previously discussed the spot film device as an addition that is installed on tables in order to execute serial radiographs, after fluoroscopic visualization of the region of interest. We are now interested in defining more precisely the functions and specific characteristics of spot films devices [5].

Spot film devices must have an electromechanical or electronic positioning system and subdivision of the images, for example, the possibility to take four consecutive images of an organ or part of or an organ on the same film. This is essential when the digestive system is being examined and the patient is given a contrast medium, such as barium, orally and the movement of the contrast medium through the esophagus, stomach, etc, needs to be observed. Taking multiple consecutive images is also used

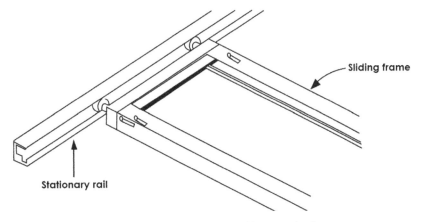

Figure 7.4. A ceiling support with external rails.

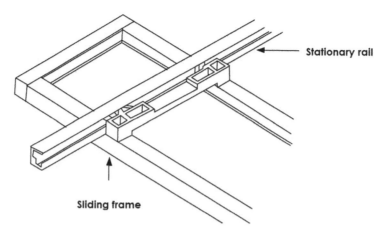

Figure 7.5. A ceiling support with internal rails.

in studies of the large intestine with barium solution dye administered rectally using an enema. Under these conditions fluoroscopy is the most effective resource, as it allows observation of the patient's body using low radiation values. This is possible through electronic systems that enhance images produced with a low dose and show the studied region on the screen of a TV monitor. Fluoroscopy also tracks the movement of the dye in the region of interest and allows the right time to make the radiographic shot to be chosen. This is the point when the spot film must switch from the fluoroscopic monitoring function to the radiographic documentation function. For this, the spot film has a manual switch in the same rack or a remote control on the floor which is operated with the foot.

The next step is to introduce, after selecting the desired subdivisions, the cassette into the path of the radiation and the patient, through an order issued by a switch on the trigger or button on the spot film device. This interrupts the fluoroscopic radiation, and once the cassette has been positioned, the radiographic shot is performed. The second shot is taken automatically after the spot film device has positioned the cassette in another sector.

It should be understood that the full surface of the film must be not impressed with the first shot. There needs to be a system of diaphragms that covers the entire cassette, except for a section that is exposed in each step of the sequence. The subsequent shots expose different sections of the film and finally the spot film device blocks the possibility of new shots, because the entire film surface has been exposed. Obviously all types of spot film devices allow the possibility to choose the shape and size of the subdivisions (two or three longitudinal, four square, or a panoramic image on the complete un-subdivided film). When more shots need to be taken, a new cassette must be inserted and the desired subdivisions reselected.

The spot film device must have the ability to manipulate the function of the fluoroscopic tube, this means that the spot film device should control the collimator. In other words it needs to be able to remotely open and close the collimator located in the tube under the table. There should be the ability to choose an automatic collimation for the selected formats or subdivisions, the choice to use different cassette sizes and the ability to easily select the diaphragm sheets in order to obtain subdivisions. Some devices have an automatic aperture with settings defined by sensors according to the size of the cassette introduced to move the laminated sheets to make them match the chosen program divisions. Other devices have laminated sheets of the required size which are inserted and removed by hand.

In terms of the spot film control brakes, the spot film device should move freely and smoothly throughout the region to be studied, but when the radiologist requires, be locked in position by means of vertical, horizontal, lateral and transverse brakes. Also, an automatic brake is activated when crossing the centered position with respect to the table. This is intended to pinpoint the midpoint of the table to use as a reference in the positioning of the TV image and the areas to consider in the patient.

Spot film devices have two methods of cassette loading. The first is top-loading, in which the cassette is inserted through the upper right-hand side of the spot film device, and is placed so that when the positioning of the cassette is selected, it goes to the left where it is located in the path of the radiation. The other method is known as lateral load in which the cassette is placed in a lateral slot near the operator so that a switch can give the order to insert to the right-hand side, in anticipation of the order to enter the field of radiation, located on the left-hand side. Figure 7.6 shows a top-loading spot film device with an image intensifier.

In addition to the laminated sheets to select the divisions, the spot film device has a removable grid for use in certain studies (see the functions of anti-scatter grids in section 7.6). Detectors for automatic dose control can also be installed. Spot film devices have the ability to position the image intensifier (which is usually installed to the left of the spot film device) at the location of the diaphragm and the mechanism of subdivision, i.e. the path of the x-rays. Spot film devices can also remove the image intensifier and install in its place a fluoroscopic screen. The latter is rarely used today.

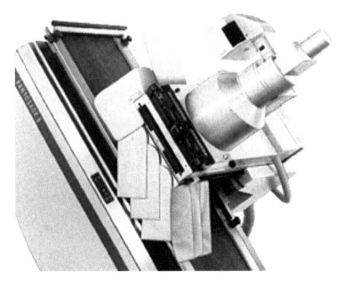

Figure 7.6. A top-loading spot film device. Courtesy of Koninklijke Philips N. V.

Another feature of spot film devices is the possibility of being mobilized by means of a motor operated from the switches installed in the spot film controller. This allows several velocities in the movement perpendicular to the patient, in particular when the table is upright. For proper positioning in any position adequate balances are required. Spot film devices can also control the tilting of the table, and the longitudinal or lateral displacement of the board on which the patient lies, so it is possible to displace the board relative to the position of the radiation beam without moving the patient in order to locate the region of study.

To achieve the required function of any spot film device, there is a delicate positioning mechanism to obtain the subdivisions, which can be more or less complex, depending on the modern technological possibilities. The most sophisticated equipment is controlled by complex electronic circuits, with extensive use of digital circuits and opto-couplers, and some devices have engines with a digital display of the sequence and subdivisions. All of these features result in relatively frequent failures of spot film devices in regular use, which necessitates appropriate use by the medical and technical staff and proper preventive maintenance.

In terms of size, specifications and cassettes, spot film devices are divided into the following types.

Accepted sizes:
- 20×24 cm^2 (8×10 inch^2)
- 24×24 cm^2 (91.2×91.2 inch^2)
- 24×30 cm^2 (10×12 inch^2)
- 30×24 cm^2 (12×10 inch^2)
- 35×35 cm^2 (14×14 inch^2)
- 28×35 cm^2 (11×14 inch^2)
- 35×43 cm^2 (14×17 inch^2)

Possible divisions of cassettes are listed in table 7.1 and shown in figure 7.7.

Finally, we note that it is important to have a high speed input of the films to facilitate studies, of the level of 0.8–1 s.

7.5 Restrictors and collimators

When an image is taken, it is necessary to expose only the region of interest, which is achieved through restriction or collimation of the radiation beam coming out of the tube. Collimation means an adjustable delimitation of the part to be irradiated to

Table 7.1. Divisions of cassettes for different sizes of film.

Film size	Formats
24×24 cm^2	1-in-1, 2-in-1, 4-in-1, 6-in-1, 9-in-1, 2-in-1
30×24 cm^2	1-in-1, 2-in-1, 4-in-1, 6-in-1, 9-in-1, 2-in-1
24×39 cm^2	1-in-1, 2-in-1
35×35 cm^2	1-in-1, 2-in-1, 3-in-1
28×35 cm^2	1-in-1, 2-in-1
35×43 cm^2	1-in-1, 2-in-1

Technical Fundamentals of Radiology and CT

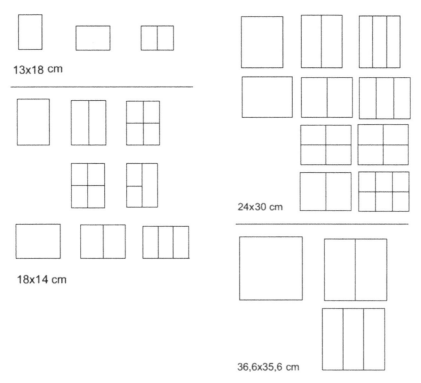

Figure 7.7. Subdivisions of images possible to obtain on the spot film device.

protect the region surrounding the organ or other body part examined. A simple form of collimation used in the most basic devices is irradiation without restriction, with sheets of shielding lead located around the irradiated body. In large-scale radiological practice other more effective and rapid methods of restriction, such as collimators, cylinders and cones, are used.

An x-ray collimator is a mechanical or electromechanical device which is more complex than cylindrical or cone restrictors.

7.5.1 Cylinder and cone restriction

A cylinder has the advantage that it can be connected directly to the tube outlet, so that it reduces the diameter of the beam and optionally can be used to immobilize the patient's head through direct contact. In studies of sinuses, some cylinders can be used connected to the output of a collimator. These cylinders have a telescopic action, i.e. they change length by displacement of one cylinder inside another, with a range of 25–50 cm. When a cylinder is connected, the radiation coming out in all directions from the tube is reduced to that which can go parallel to the cylinder walls. The rest of the radiation bundle crashes into the walls of the tube which absorb the radiation because they contain sheets of lead. Thus the incident x-rays strike only the region which delimits the cylinder and also absorbs any form of scattered radiation which may be created by impacts on the region to be radiographed.

Technical Fundamentals of Radiology and CT

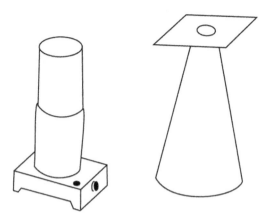

Figure 7.8. Example of cylinder and cone restrictors.

Projection cones also produce the same effect with the difference that the radiation is divergent, so that a cone can move with the tube relative to the patient to modify the diameter of the region to be radiographed, respecting the distance range tube–film as it is normed (100–183 cm). Figure 7.8 shows drawings of a cylinder with its latching mechanism to the tube and a cone restrictor.

7.5.2 Collimators

One of the most important accessories used in radiology is the collimator. Its function is to provide a variable adjustment of the surface to be irradiated. Collimators can be rectangular or ring-shaped (an 'iris' collimator). Rectangular collimators consist of horizontal and vertical blades that can be adjusted independently, so as to control the dimensions of the rectangle separately in both directions. Iris collimators always open or close a circle of variable diameter. Such collimators are used in special applications, in particular with devices attached to TV systems.

The collimators can be manually operated or motorized. Manually operated collimators are usually used in x-ray tubes mounted on floor–wall or floor–ceiling stands, so that the operator can adjust the collimator according to their needs, usually so that the radiation beam matches the dimensions of the standard sized film cassette. To determine the dimensions of the radiation beam and the position of the tube relative to the patient, the collimator has a bulb from which intense light is projected onto a mirror positioned in such a way that it illuminates the object to be x-rayed with the same projection as the output of the x-ray beam. The radiation can pass through without altering the mirror located on its trajectory. All this is clearly shown in figure 7.9.

Motorized collimators [6] have a pair of motors that are responsible for moving the diaphragms by means of gears and suitable transmissions, similarly to manually operated collimators. Such devices are generally used in fluoroscopic tubes under tables and due to their applications it is unnecessary to equip them with a light. The remote control of the movement and action of the collimator diaphragms occurs through the controls located on the spot film device and is controlled by an operator using an image on a TV monitor.

Collimators have some attachments that simplify the technical work of the operator, such as a distance meter which is used to correctly position the patient relative to the tube. A tape measure wrapped around the cabinet of the collimator is also used to measure the distance from the tube to the patient in a wall holder system. The collimator has filters composed of aluminum sheets of different thicknesses [7] to filter low energy radiation that does not improve the radiographic image and avoid exposing the patient to unnecessary radiation.

Some types of collimators have a graduated scale or digital display (see figure 7.10) indicating the technical dimension of the rectangle, which corresponds to certain

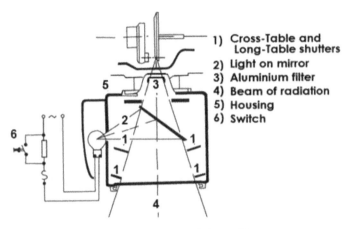

Figure 7.9. A manual multiplane collimator.

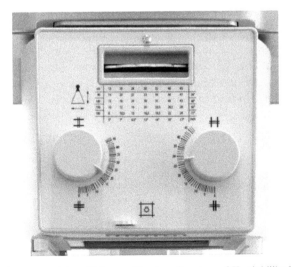

Figure 7.10. A commercial multiplane collimator. Courtesy of Koninklijke Philips N. V.

formats of cassettes. This indication is essential when, for some reason, there is no light collimator. Brake controls are located on the collimator handlebars to obtain the correct positioning and angle of the tube on the column stand.

7.6 Anti-scatter grids

In 1913 Dr Gustav Bucky created the diaphragm type grid, an anti-scatter placed between the patient and the film, in order to eliminate the secondary radiation that impresses the film deforming the image and reducing its diagnostic value. This grid allows radiation to reach the film from the tube [8], but absorbs rebounding radiation coming from the patient's body, i.e. secondary or scattered radiation which reaches the film with a different angle of incidence.

The resulting advantage is significant because it reduces deformation and thus solved a fundamental problem in radiology. However, a new problem arose, namely the appearance of the projected grid on the film generating a shadow. Dr Hollis Potter invented a method of moving the grid during exposure, so that its projected image is blurred on the film. The Potter–Bucky grid system, which is considered to be essential in all current radiological installations, became commercially available in 1920. The full anti-scatter system, including the grid, the mechanism that moves during radiation, the tray and the cassette holder, is known as the Bucky system.

7.6.1 Grids

A grid is a component of the anti-scatter system whose function is to filter unwanted radiation. It consists of a series of staggered strips of translucent material and lead strips. The translucent material is called the window, and can be made of plastic, magnesium, balsa wood, or aluminum. The number of lead strips defines the capacity of the grid to eliminate secondary radiation, which is measured by the so-called grid ratio and the number of strips of lead per centimeter. Thus a grid with a low grating ratio, but with a large number of lead strips per centimeter, will be as effective as a grid with a high ratio but fewer strips of lead per centimeter.

The grid ratio is defined as the ratio between the length of a strip of lead and the length of the space between two strips, as shown in figure 7.11. Accordingly, a grid relationship of 8:1 means that the height or length of the lead strips is eight times greater than the distance between the strips or, equivalently, is eight times greater than the width of the window material used to support the lead strips.

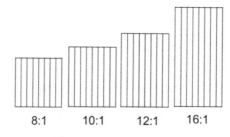

Figure 7.11. Grid relations.

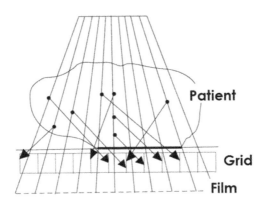

Figure 7.12. The function of a grid.

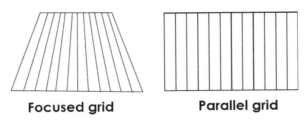

Figure 7.13. Two types of grids.

Figure 7.12 shows the process of removing unwanted radiation from impacting on the film. The primary x-ray beam passes through the patient's body, casting its shadow over the film, while rays arising from scattering, with different angles of incidence, are overridden by the strips of lead.

Using gratings with a high grid ratio [9] is advisable in circumstances where the distance between the grid and the film is fixed, and in cases where the automatic centering of the tube is easily performed. In other cases the use of grids with a lower ratio is recommended.

7.6.2. Types of grids

Grids are manufactured in three different forms (see figure 7.13): parallel, focused and grating grids. Parallel grids are used when the distance between the tube and the grid is large, so that the primary radiation that reaches the grid can pass through without being blocked by strips of lead. If the grid is near the tube, not much radiation can pass through, particularly in regions far from the center.

Focused grids have a divergent arrangement of the lead strips to the film and a convergent arrangement towards the tube, so that the primary radiation can always pass through the strips at lower grid–tube distances than for the parallel grid.

Gridded grids are used for specialized studies in which tubes are used with a constant distance relative to the grid. Since such grids must be carefully aligned with regard to the beam, to avoid cutting the edges off the radiation, the tube must be

Technical Fundamentals of Radiology and CT

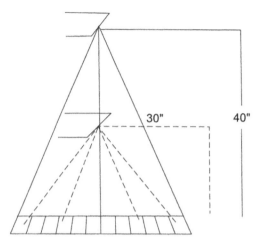

Figure 7.14. . Grid radius or focal length.

perfectly perpendicular to the grid and the patient must also be carefully positioned. Despite all these drawbacks, this type of grid is best to avoid the fogging effects of high radiation levels on the image of the film.

7.6.3 Grid connection and focal length

A grid's focus should be defined depending on the focal length or radius of the grid, which is the distance between the grid and the point at which the lead strips converge (see figure 7.14). This means that if this distance is not taken into account, the primary radiation will be absorbed by the lead sheet, reducing the radiographic efficacy of the shot.

Focused grids have radii of 92, 102, 122, 153 and 183 cm. Unfocused grids should not be located within a distance of less than 92 cm from the anode, because the primary radiation reduction would be unacceptable. The number of lead strips by grid, i.e. the number of lines per cm, must have a maximum of 100, grids commonly in use have 20 or 24 lines per cm as the most acceptable values.

Also important is the angle at which the x-rays are incident on the grid; there is a relationship between this angle and the grid ratio. If the grid ratio is higher, the radiation beam can only have smaller angles of incidence, this is shown in figure 7.15. The strips or sheets should be placed parallel to the length of the radiographic table, i.e. along the length of the patient.

7.6.4 Grid movement

The grid can be moved by two basic mechanisms. The first is called simple hit, in which, using a mechanical or an electromagnetic relay system, the grid is hit at a specific moment, so as to move and return via some elastic strip or spring. These systems are manually loaded and activated by the operator to move them along the patient in a perpendicular direction. The duration of movement can be selected. The minimum allowable exposure time is 1/20 s and the mechanism must be mounted so

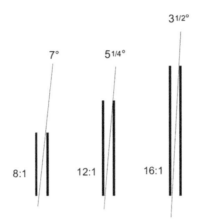

Figure 7.15. The angle of incidence and grid connection.

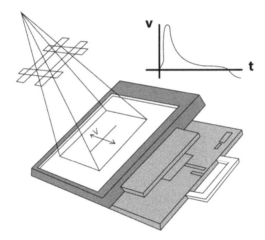

Figure 7.16. The movement of an anti-scatter grid.

that the grid movement starts before the radiation. The displacement time of the grid should be such that it does not end before the radiation ends.

The second type of grid movement is achieved through what is known as a reciprocating system. A motor controls forward and backward movement of the film. In this case the travel time of the grid and its speed cannot be adjusted by the operator, requiring additional irradiation times of at least a quarter of a second. If this movement of the grid is not fast enough it cannot prevent the grid strips from projecting their shadow onto the film. In the rest position the grid is somewhat offset from the center of radiation so that the movement begins before the exposure. The focus is achieved during the motion of the grid, otherwise the grid would be outside the center with the corresponding radiation loss and the appearance of lines on the film. This explains the need for a minimum radiation time in the use of such grids. Figure 7.16 shows the curve produced by the movement of an anti-scatter grid in time.

References

[1] General Electric Medical Systems 1983 Introduction to radiographic equipment *Training Course*

[2] General Electric Medical Systems 1977 Soporte mural Bucky *Product Data* 1704

[3] Siemens 1989 Estativo de columna U con guías de suelo techo *Installation Manual* R21-020031040107

[4] Universal Allied Imaging 1999 Pulsar medical system *Catalog* 070184

[5] General Electric Medical Systems 1986 RFX model 11 spotfilmer *Product Data* B8415

[6] Klemm T 1969 El nuevo colimador multiplano *Rev. SRW* **1** 6–9

[7] The Machlett Lab 1999 Duocon M, manual collimator *Technical Manual* ST 3252

[8] Goel A *et al* Grids *Radiopaedia* http://radiopaedia.org/articles/grids accessed 2015

[9] Anderson D W 2006 Introduction of grids to mobile ICU radiography in a teaching hospital *Br. J. Radiol.* **5** 315–8

IOP Publishing

Technical Fundamentals of Radiology and CT

Guillermo Avendaño Cervantes

Chapter 8

Automatic exposure control

8.1 Introduction

For a good radiograph one needs to select the appropriate kVp, tube current and time of exposure. Many devices have established current values so only the kVp and time need to be selected, some equipment works selecting only a percentage, others selecting the desired current and exposure time, and some selecting only the kVp. Whatever the mode selected, it is clear that with a high volume of patients it is necessary to invest a lot of time in determining these values, which can lead to errors or excessive delays. One must also consider the individual patient anatomy and pathology. This is why the so-called automatic exposure control (AEC), or automatic dose system, for radiation was created [1].

The basic function of an AEC system is determining the duration of a radiographic exposure and is based on achieving a certain level of radiation on the patient. During exposure of the film, the radiation is measured by an instrument that compares the values with previously established parameters, so that when the desired value is reached, the radiation is interrupted by an order from the same instrument.

Currently three systems are used, ionization chambers, photoelectric systems and solid-state radiation detectors (SSRDs). Using these systems of AEC a large volume of images can be obtained with good radiographic quality over a shorter time. In ionization chambers, a photomultiplier tube is sandwiched between the patient and the film. It is a special ionization sensor [2] that does not alter the path of or absorb the radiation, but is capable of measuring the amount of radiation and giving the interrupt signal.

Photoelectric systems are based on the illumination of a fluorescent screen by radiation which has already passed through the patient and activates a photo-multiplier which releases an amount of current proportional to the light. When the preselected value is reached exposure interruption occurs.

doi:10.1088/978-0-7503-1212-7ch8   8-1   © IOP Publishing Ltd 2016

SSRDs are placed behind the film. The current of the SSRD is proportional to the dose rate behind the cassette and not to that in the plane of the film, so the optical density is no longer proportional to the detector current.

8.2 Ionization chambers

The first ionization chamber system was invented by Leo Szilard and is based on the measurement of air ionization. The key component of this system is the ionization chamber, a device that is inserted in the path of the radiation that crosses the body of the patient and the film. Its function is to measure the ionization of the air contained in the chamber caused by the x-rays passing through it.

The ionization chamber produces a change in its internal resistance in response to the ionization, such that it acts as a variable resistor in series with a capacitor which determines the charging voltage which activates a relay cutting the radiation [3]. The higher the radiation dose is, the faster the trigger voltage is reached. This device has a resistance–capacitance time constant given by the capacity value and the variable resistor of the ionization chamber.

The ionization chamber should be as narrow as possible and should not create any shadows on the film. It is formed by two outer layers of Mylar that act as plastic covers, containing electrodes called emitters which receive the x-rays without affecting them, but achieve ionization of the air and create electrons projected on the collectors, which have a voltage of about 300 V with respect to the emitters. It is clear that when there are more x-rays more secondary electrons are created, drastically reducing the resistance between the emitters and collectors. There is a translucent material on both sides of the emitter and the collector, and between them is the air that will be ionized by the x-rays (see figure 8.1.).

The ionization chamber is a variable resistor with a capacitor that is connected in series, and a continuous charging voltage is applied over both. On the arrival of x-rays, the air in the gap changes from infinite resistance to a value that produces a charge in the capacitor. According to the dose of x-rays obtained with a given voltage, the silicon-controlled rectifier (SCR) is activated, driving the response to interrupt radiation.

The basic circuit shown in figure 8.2 is used in some commercial devices, however, modern electronic sophistication has led to highly accurate, complex devices that produce remarkable results. X-ray devices generally use three ionization chambers covering the whole area to be explored. One of these is called the dominant chamber, which is chosen according to the type of study to be carried out. In a radiograph the dominant region should maintain a specific average optical density. Thus AEC systems are suitable for all types of exposures where the equipment allows alignment of the measuring field and dominant region, and where the collimated x-ray field of exposure is not smaller than the measuring field [4].

Technical Fundamentals of Radiology and CT

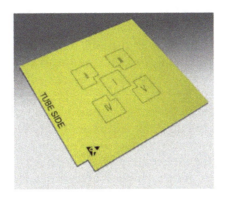

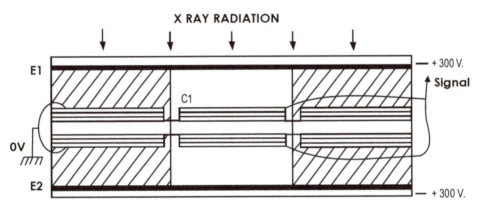

Figure 8.1. The structure of an ionization chamber.

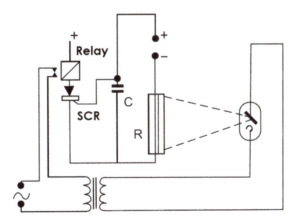

Figure 8.2. An exposure meter within an ionization chamber.

8.3 Photoelectric systems

Photoelectric exposure meters are based on the formation of a fluoroscopic image on a screen and the use of the image brightness to activate the timer. In the chain of electronic components that make up such a system, one is a fundamental element, the photomultiplier tube. This tube converts the incident radiation passing through the patient into light, then generates electrons according the level of light created. Photomultiplier tubes have numerous electrodes to produce an increased number of electrons. The resultant current is proportional to the incident brightness and is the parameter that governs the interruption of shooting.

Not all the components of these systems are translucent to x-rays, so they cannot be placed in the radiation beam. The photomultiplier tubes are installed behind the patient and behind the film, so are not affected by filtration changes, density changes or changing the distance from the patient to the film.

Exposure meters (see figure 8.3) based on photoelectric systems can be implemented in two ways:

1. Using a container for the screen and the photomultiplier behind the patient. The container is a dark chamber. When it receives x-rays the fluorescent screen lights up and the light is amplified by the photomultiplier. The radiographic film cassette is installed in front of the screen and can be easily loaded.
2. By means of an image intensifier system (see figure 8.4), similar to that used in the fluoroscopic screen, but many times greater in intensity. This image created on the secondary screen of the intensifier is projected onto a set of optical lenses, which carry the image on the photomultiplier to a large format camera. The image can also be switched through a mirror into a TV camera or radiographic film. The photomultiplier installed on the side of the camera collects light proportional to the radiation and triggers charging of the shooting capacitor.

Photomultiplier tubes (see figure 8.5) can be constructed based on ladder or ring electrodes, in both the basis of operation is the same. When light falls on the cathode

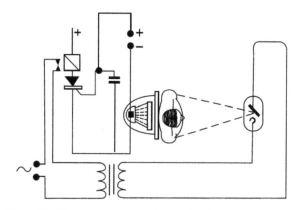

Figure 8.3. The exposure meter circuit of a photoelectric system.

Technical Fundamentals of Radiology and CT

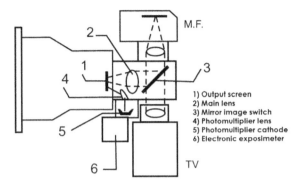

Figure 8.4. An exposure meter image intensifier.

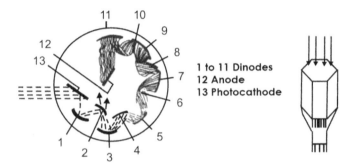

Figure 8.5. A photomultiplier tube.

of the tube, emission of electrons is generated. These are attracted to specific electrodes (called dynodes). The electrons produced can only reach the dynodes along a specific path. The voltage of each dynode is increased and the impact of electrons on each dynode releases a lot of secondary electrons, which are directed in turn to the next dynode, so that a cumulative effect is produced and each dynode releases a larger number of electrons. Finally with significant amplification, the electrons impact on the anode, producing an amount of electric charge which becomes a current sufficiently high to load the capacitor that controls the radiographic shot. This system must be mounted on the photomultiplier side and with the possibility to be removed for replacement if necessary.

Practical circuits of automatic dose control [2] contain components such as operational amplifiers and multi-turn potentiometers that achieve fine adjustment of radiographic shot times depending on the desired dose.

8.4 SSRDs

SSRDs are highly sensitive to the dose. They are highly integrated electronic circuits which directly generate an electrical signal proportional to the level of radiation [5] (see figure 8.6). This type of detector is perfectly adequate for devices where lower dose

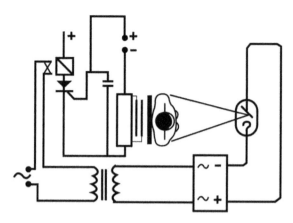

Figure 8.6. An SSRD system.

levels are used, such as those used in pediatrics and mammography. The advantage of SSRDs over ionization chambers is that the dose can be kept somewhat lower due to reduced absorption in front of the film.

References

[1] Szasz S 1977 Automatic dose rate control and its application *Medicor News* **2** 30–40
[2] Komiathy I 1977 Application of automatic exposure timer (type res II) with Medicor x-ray equipment *Medicor News* **2** 68–76
[3] General Electric Medical Systems 1987 Quantamat *Service Manual*
[4] General Electric Medical Systems 1988 Introducing MSX *Catalog* OM 0304
[5] Elderyi M 1973 Medical experiences with the x-ray generator EDR-750 *Medicor News* **3** 6–10

IOP Publishing

Technical Fundamentals of Radiology and CT

Guillermo Avendaño Cervantes

Chapter 9

Film changer

9.1 Introduction

So far we have studied devices that can use a cassette with radiographic film that is exposed in full (panoramic mode) or can be divided into several sections or parts (2, 3, 4 or 8). We have described simple systems in which the process is controlled through the intervention of the technician using the collimator and changing the cassette position, which allows arbitrary divisions of the film. Spot film devices can make this whole process automated, allowing different formats, such as those detailed in chapter 7.

In actual radiological practice it is important to produce a very fast set of x-rays images that serve to study continuous phenomena in time, such as the vessels of the heart or brain filled with blood, peripheral circulatory or digestive system functions, etc. In such cases additional equipment is needed to quickly switch the film in the path of the x-rays, so that films can be exposed in rapid sequence. If these film changers can meet a set of technical requirements, they will be a very useful radiological accessory.

The most commonly used film changer is loaded with a high number of films of the same format. Using a delicate electromechanical system, the film is inserted in the path of the radiation and removed quickly once it has been exposed. This type of changer handles the entire process in a virtual dark room and allows the removal of films from the changer once full, without affecting the films.

There are also more complex and expensive systems that work without radiographic cassette equipment, namely, through a changer joined to the device. After exposure the films are moved to a certain point where the film is revealed without leaving the device. Due to the fact these devices are not in widespread used, they will not be discussed further in this book.

The universally known systems are the AOT system and a device called PUCK [1]. The latter comes in two versions, U-shaped, which is used for pure radiography studies, and L-shaped, which is used when fluoroscopy and radiography are required

doi:10.1088/978-0-7503-1212-7ch9   9-1   © IOP Publishing Ltd 2016

simultaneously. Although the PUCK system and its name correspond to a product of a particular commercial company (as does AOT), the use of these systems is widespread in different devices from various companies, and the terms have become generic. For this reason we refer to both the AOT and PUCK systems with their proper names.

9.2 The AOT system

The AOT system consists of a bulky but mobile cabinet, which contains a complex system of gears and rollers designed to make the mechanism withdraw one unexposed film at a time from a container and place it in a position perpendicular to the radiation (see figure 9.1). Then the film is introduced to another container where the exposed films are accumulated. Its dimensions make it suitable for positioning close to the patient to avoid distortion of the image.

The displacement of the film is circular, the film starts its motion when is removed by extraction pawls and it is then positioned in the right place by rollers, so that it is in the path of the x-rays. Once exposed, it is moved down where it is received in a container called the cassette (equivalent to a darkroom). This process is repeated for as many films as necessary. When all the films have been exposed, the device can disengage both the container and the tank of exposed films, known as the cassette; to recharge the former and to reveal the contents of the other.

The cabinet of the electromechanical system is governed by a control that serves to program the sequence of the films, that is, the rate at which they are exposed, the time interval between films, etc. It can also be programmed to expose a single film. The control of a changer must be sufficiently reliable to function alongside the x-ray generator during the programmed sequence that determines the respective radiographic shot.

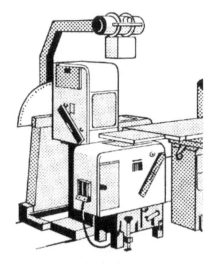

Figure 9.1. A double AOT system.

9.3 The PUCK system

The PUCK film changer system (see figure 9.2) is governed by a control [2] that allows work programs to be developed through using a punch card. Using such controls the procedure is selected for singular shot or a preset sequence. This sequence corresponds to the number and frequency of films to be exposed for the purpose of documenting a certain type of study. The start trigger is controlled by a manual button attached to the control.

The punch card is programmed manually [3] and contains the various possible combinations for shots, i.e., the number of films per second, the stop order and orders to command the action of the contrast medium injector, which administers the substances at the appropriate moment that the system requires. The card is also programmed to control the movements of the examination table when it is also directed by the changer control system. So we have, for example, a sequence of two exposures per second for three seconds, three exposures per second for five seconds and one exposure per second for six seconds; this allows us to calculate the sequence and the total time used. This is in the first line of the card, which is a timeline. In the second line we include stop orders for each sequence before starting the next. The third and fourth lines consider the movements of the table forward or backward, respectively.

The holder for programmed punch cards is located in the control panel, along with the respective reader, which is provided with LEDs paired with

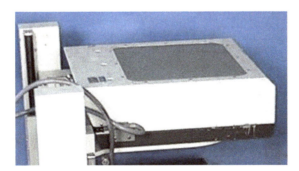

Figure 9.2. A horizontal PUCK changer. Courtesy of Siemens.

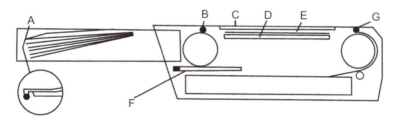

Figure 9.3. The internal structure of a PUCK changer. Courtesy of Siemens.

phototransistors and switches that select the type of work to be done. The control panel also has a timer with a switch to start the sequence of work and an emergency stop switch to abort the process in case of any anomaly.

PUCK systems can also have a control system based on a microprocessor which gives more versatility in programming and other system capabilities. This method, which is more advanced than the punch card system, allows the operator to perform corrections in programming, storing up to 19 program sequences appropriate for specific organs, etc. The system has the possibility of using a control console arranged on a pedestal, according to local conditions [4]. The console has a keyboard and corresponding illuminated keys that allow proper operation. There are also system changers manufactured by CANON and Compagnie Generale de Radiologie.

Figure 9.3 shows the internal structure of a PUCK type film changer. The film loader [5] (magazine) shows the pawl in the film conveyor (A). The film is pushed into the exchanger through the inlet compressor roller (B). The film is positioned between sheets (C) and (D), which has an intensifying screen (E). After being exposed to the x-rays, the film passes through the compressor roller (G), where it is curved against a larger roller and deposited in the output bin or cassette. F indicates the cylinder where the patient name is located.

References

[1] Foster E 1985 *Equipment for Diagnostic Radiography* (London: Springer)

[2] Siemens-Elema AB 1987 Puck film changer units *Service Manual*

[3] Holik B 1977 Método para evitar la programación errónea en la angiografía de la pelvis y pierna con desplazamiento por pasos del tablero de mesa *Electromédica* **2** 45–51

[4] Crolla D, Baert L and Romhildt K 1979 Routine magnification angiography using the PUCK 24 or AOT-35 outfilm changer and the optilix 110/12/50 HSG microfocus x-ray tube *Electromédica* **3** 89–97

[5] Siemens-Elema AB 1986 PUCK Blattfilmwechsler *Data* MR 33/7027

IOP Publishing

Technical Fundamentals of Radiology and CT

Guillermo Avendaño Cervantes

Chapter 10

Cinefluorography systems

10.1 Introduction

Fluoroscopy is commonly used in various diagnostic procedures. It is of prime importance in angiographic studies (see figure 10.1), where it is a priority to have excellent contrast of blood vessels and also a very good resolution for close observation of fine vascularization [1]. Catheterization of any blood vessel, in particular those related to the heart and brain, must be performed accurately and with appropriate levels of radiation [2].

Interventional angiography for diagnostic or therapeutic (implanted pacemaker or angioplasty) purposes [3] needs to be carried out under the safest possible conditions. Safety relates to the perfect delineation of borders and the exact location of each vessel branch, as the catheter must be tracked through tortuous vessels.

So it follows that the quality of imaging systems is vital for this type of work. Fluoroscopic systems combined with cine film [4] allow images to be obtained with an adequate quality for the purposes required, provided that the complete system of components does not contain any inappropriate parts. As a full system will not work if it has a faulty part, in practical terms this is equivalent to having a completely damaged system.

The output of the fluoroscopic TV, whether for film or video recorded on tape, must be of high resolution, so that smearing of the image is avoided and proper contrast is obtained. At the same time, the system must not be saturated when certain regions of low absorption are irradiated. Moreover, despite the low levels of radiation, the system must be able to provide information in the form of good images for all patients [5], regardless of their thickness. Finally, the system should automatically be set to obtain the best possible image without operator intervention

10.2 The components of a cinefluorographic system

All cinefluorographic systems consist of the following components:
- A special x-ray tube.
- An image intensifier.

doi:10.1088/978-0-7503-1212-7ch10   10-1   © IOP Publishing Ltd 2016

- An optical coupler.
- A system for radiographic film.
- A system for radiological TV.
- Components for recording.
- A digitizer for DSA.

Among all the different components of the fluoroscopic system, we will focus on the electronic function of the cine and TV systems, consisting of a set of specialized components and circuitry to achieve high quality images with a high degree of automation. Figure 10.2 shows the general components of a system for TV images

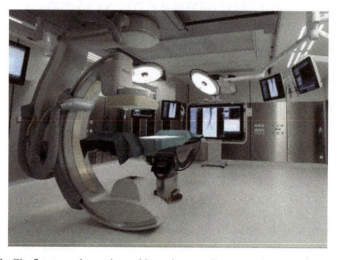

Figure 10.1. Cinefluorography angiographic equipment. Courtesy of Koninklijke Philips N. V.

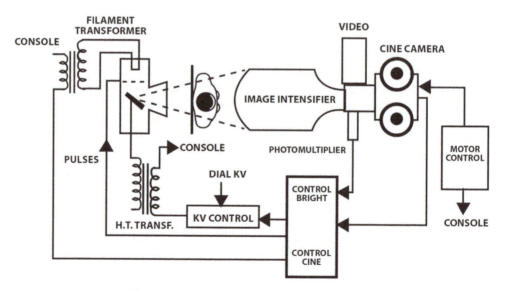

Figure 10.2. A diagram of a fluoroscopic TV system.

and radiographic film. We can see that the signals of the automatic brightness control and cine pulses modify the values of kVp and filament current (acting over mA), so that the radiation is automatically adjusted to the best level for filming and for the video image

To see the heart in real time, it is necessary that sequential images are obtained with a frequency that gives a sense of continuity. Physiologically, this is called the fusion frequency, the frequency at which images are fused without intervals in the retina of the viewer. This means a range of 30–90 images per second. The radiation applied in cardiac studies cannot last more than 5 ms in adults and 3 ms in children.

To obtain penetrating x-rays regardless of the morphology of the patient, the device should have a tube up to 120 kV and a level of radiation that allows the visualization of vessels with contrast. Therefore, a compromise must be made between the level of radiation that, of course, may not be very high, and the minimum detectable dose for the desired contrast. Thus, the tube must be able to supply between 20–40 mR for cine pictures with an image intensifier of 15 cm.

The way to achieve this is by controlling the emission of x-rays. The tube must have the appropriate focal spot to achieve the desired resolution (a small focus). The tube used in these devices needs to have a particularly good heat dissipation capacity of the anode and rapid cooling time in order not to limit the rate of study (the frequency of patients examined).

To obtain shorter exposure times and at the same time a high frequency of images per second, it is necessary to control the emission in the tube itself, through a polarized grid that governs the radiation, blocking emission of x-rays when the potential applied to it is negative and permitting emission when there is no tension. This way has two main advantages: the radiation is reduced to half of what the patient would receive with continuous operation of the radiation, and the tube life time is significantly extended, since it only radiates when the control pulse gives the command. Control by means of a grid has the additional advantage that in pediatric applications it can achieve pulses as short as 25 ms, which are impossible to achieve by other methods. The tubes should have two focal spots, one produced by a large focus for adult applications and another small focus spot to provide lower emission, generally intended for use in fluoroscopy and pediatric work.

10.3 Radiological TV systems

Incorporating radiological TV has meant a revolutionary change in certain diagnostic procedures, because it has allowed the possibility of real-time tests and complete examination prior to radiographic documentation. Before the appearance of x-ray TV, exploration studies on fluoroscopic screens had the disadvantages of limited brightness of images and excessive radiation exposure to the operator. Moreover, without a mechanism to increase the intensity of the brightness of the screen, it was not possible to install a TV camera. Therefore, the introduction of image intensification systems has led to an adequate standard of luminous intensity for a TV camera and a corresponding process can be adapted for fluoroscopic systems. Figure 10.3 shows a comparison between light that reaches the human eye in a screen system and an image intensifier system, and allows us to assess the importance of achieving a better image with lower levels of radiation.

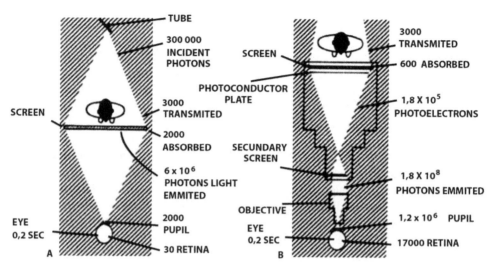

Figure 10.3. Comparison between a screen system and an image intensifier system.

10.3.1 X-ray TV

A radiological TV system consists of the following components:
- A fluoroscopic radiation generator.
- An image intensifier.
- A TV camera with a pick up tube.
- A TV center.
- A TV monitor.

We will describe each component of the system separately and also discuss their interconnection with other components, including all closed loop forming elements from the tube to the monitor. The doctor should be considered as an integral part of the loop, looking at the image and feeding back the information to modify the parameters of the image obtained with the explicit purpose of improving it depending on their specific interest. Thus he/she can change the brightness, contrast, kVp and the intensity of the fluoroscopic current to achieve the central aim of observing a good image that has diagnostic value.

10.4 The fluoroscopy generator

For the system to work, there must obviously be a generator of radiation, in this case a low-level radiation or fluoroscopic source so that it can be applied for a considerably longer duration than the longest radiographic exposure times [6]. As we know, the tube intended for this purpose is called a fluoroscopic tube, and is located under the table in conventional systems.

Radiation from the tube passes through the patient and reaches the spot film device where the image intensifier or the fluoroscopy screen is mounted. In the latter case the system terminates there, as it is on the screen that the image is formed and where the doctor observes the region to study directly. To increase the intensity of the light, either the radiation through the filament current or the voltage applied to the tube is increased. When an image intensifier is used, the situation is different because the radiation levels required for the system to generate an image with adequate visibility are very low compared to previous systems.

10.5 The image intensifier

The image intensifier is similar in shape to a bottle with standardized dimensions and shape. Lenses are installed at the narrow end which allow the output image to be adapted to the pick-up TV camera, and the wider end receives radiation directly from the x-ray tube. The high vacuum tube processes the incident light from one end, turning it into electrons and reconverting the image at the other end. This process allows an output image to be obtained that is equal to the input but more intense, with a significant gain of brightness, allowing a pick-up camera to be engaged, which collects and processes this signal as video information [7]. The sequence that follows is similar to that in any transmission of CCTV.

An image intensifier consists of the following components:
- A graphite coated glass vial with a high vacuum.
- An entry screen (or the primary).
- A photocathode.
- Electrostatic focalizers.
- An anode accelerator.
- An output screen (or the secondary).
- Shielding.

As shown in figure 10.4 the image obtained can be seen directly on the secondary display [2] by means of suitable optical lenses; it is common to adapt a TV camera. We will discuss in detail the components of image intensifiers. These devices require the application of a high electric potential between the cathode and the anode photoelectric accelerator, therefore a voltage power supply is an additional necessary component for the system to work.

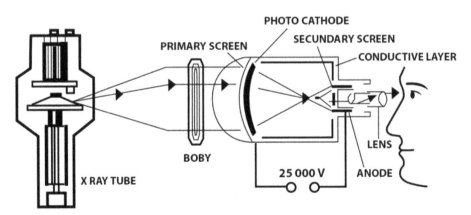

Figure 10.4. A diagram showing the principle of the image intensifier.

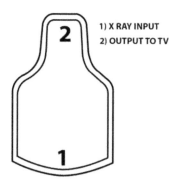

Figure 10.5. The basic structure of a glass ampoule.

10.5.1 The glass ampoule

The intensifier consists of a high vacuum tube containing the other elements. The tube is bottle-shaped and cylindrical with a narrowing at the output end, as shown in figure 10.5. As with any container that is to be under a vacuum, the glass walls must be strong enough to withstand the pressure gradient, and also sufficiently tough to withstand the movements and the tapping to which it is subjected when in use. The potential risk remains of an implosion due to defects in manufacturing or sudden drops or blows, hence it is recommended that image intensifiers are manipulated with caution and protection is used for the eyes and hands.

The ampoule is formed of glass containing graphite, whose function in shielding and blackening of the system is equivalent to a darkroom. Moreover, measures are taken to prevent magnetic fields, including the Earth's magnetic field [8], affecting the ampoules. These shields are usually metal plates covering the glass surface with a greater shielding effect for magnetic fields perpendicular to the tube axis.

10.5.2 The primary or input screen

The input screen is the most important intensifier component because this is where the conversion of one energy form to another occurs. The photons of x-rays are converted into light photons, i.e. a shift occurs in the electromagnetic spectrum from a wavelength of 40–0.01 Å (x-rays) to 4000–5000 Å (visible light).

The conversion process in x-ray luminosity is achieved through the use of various types of chemical salts of zinc, cadmium and cesium, which are basic materials to produce fluorescence [9]. Initially zinc and cadmium sulfide were used, but subsequently improved performance was achieved with cesium iodide. Obviously, work is ongoing to improve the chemicals used to provide a better substrate for conversion factors.

The input screen has the form of a specific curve following the form of the image intensifier entrance, in order to obtain sphericity to allow the convergence of the electrons produced in the photocathode, which also has the same shape.

10.5.3 The photocathode

This curvature of this element follows that of the fluorescent screen, so that they always maintain the same curvature and remain parallel with respect to each other

Technical Fundamentals of Radiology and CT

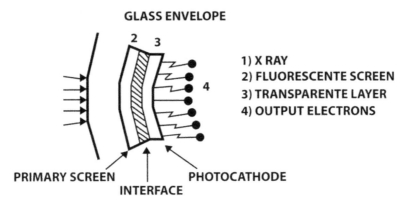

Figure 10.6. The photocathode

[10] (see figure 10.6). Thus the package of light photons produced on impact with the photocathode screen produces electrons, directly proportional in magnitude to the light generated, i.e. also in direct proportion to the x-rays.

10.5.4 Focusers

A set of electrostatic grids, located along the tube so as to cause a convergence of the electrons produced, is responsible for producing the lens effect, similar to the optical lenses of a camera. The electrons generated in the photocathode, accelerated by the high voltage, are directed to the output screen, focused by the set of said grids with voltages and a suitable physical form, thus the overall image produced in the primary display is transferred via an electronic output route to the screen [11]. The electron beam thus travels along most of the length of the glass tube, with a crossing point region where the image is reversed, placing the image on the screen in the same way as an image is formed on the film of a conventional photography camera. The grids are important due to the fact that their construction and careful polarization allow an optimal approach since each point of the input screen image must move towards the output screen without distortion [12].

10.5.5 The anode accelerator

The anode accelerator receives an application of high voltage with positive polarity and its function is to guide the electrons at the end of their journey to the output screen [13], so that they exactly cover all of its dimensions. This is achieved by giving the anode a characteristic L-shape, with the result that the greatest attraction of the electrons is at the narrowest part of the L where the electrons agglomerate [14] and are then spread to the screen by the effect of the rest of the L-shape (see figure 10.7).

10.6 The TV center

The TV center is a set of electronic circuits that takes the signal from the image capturing tube [15] (Vidicon, Hivicon, Szicon, CCD systems, etc) and processes it, so that the most appropriate image for presentation is sent to the monitor. The function of the TV center [16] is also to relate the brightness of the image with the radiation

Technical Fundamentals of Radiology and CT

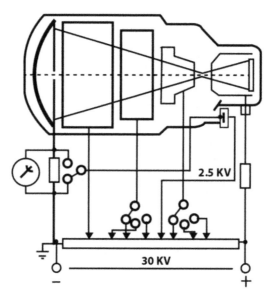

Figure 10.7. Focusers and the anode accelerator.

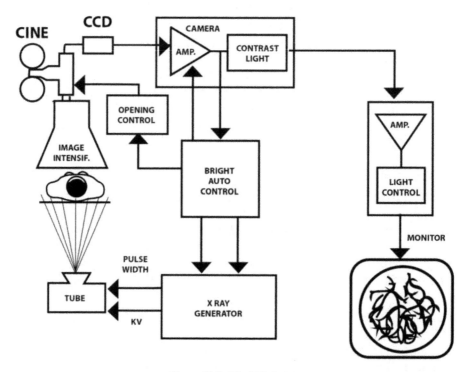

Figure 10.8. The TV chain.

incident on the patient, so that it can feed back information to the fluoroscopy generator in order to automatically adjust the values of mA and kV depending on the image on the monitor. In other words, the automatic brightness control on the monitor image also changes the fluoroscopic radiation without operator intervention [17]. The TV center contains circuits forming an electronic circle surrounding the image and adjusting the amplification of video levels and other parameters of the signal sent to the monitor. The circuit of figure 10.8 shows a block diagram of the TV chain with the set of blocks of the central TV [18].

10.7 The TV monitor

The standard signal is displayed on the monitor (see figure 10.9) which allows the physician to observe with good resolution the patient body that is being irradiated. It is also included in the system for recording video images using magnetic tape or discs [19], as shown in figure 10.10.

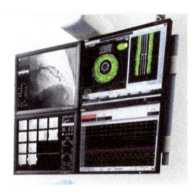

Figure 10.9. A radiological monitor. Courtesy of Siemens.

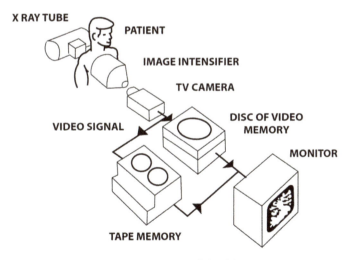

Figure 10.10. Components of the video system.

References

[1] Bischoff K 1964 La radiotelevisión se abre camino *Rev. SRW* **2** 54–9

[2] Heinkel K and Fink W 1970 Control radiológico por televisión en la aplicación de un neumoperitoneo *Rev. SRW* **3** 76–80

[3] Dunisch O and Dorr H 1969 Nuestro nuevo sistema intensificador de imagen con televisión *Rev. SRW* **1** 14–9

[4] Kruger W 1973 Una moderna instalación de TV radiológica *Med. Technik* B **1** 12–6

[5] General Electric Medical Systems 1983 Image intensification and recording devices *Training Course*

[6] Sturmer W 1969 La conversión de imágenes por medio de semiconductores *Rev. SRW* **2** 6–8

[7] Princot J and Niepel J 1978 Indirect radiographic technique using the Sircam cammeras and an x-ray image intensifier in radiology of the digestive tract *Electromedica* **2** 60–4

[8] Haendle J, Horbaschek H and Alesandrescu M 1977 La roentgentelevisión de alta resolución y las memorias de video de alta resolución *Electromedica* **1** 12–9

[9] Pujadas G, Garlando C, Tamasiho A and Florm C 1977 El uso de la cineradiografía en la arteriografía periférica *Electromedica* **2** 27–32

[10] Siemens 1998 Equipo intensificador de imagen y roentgentelevisión *Information for Medical Technicians*

[11] Gudden F 1981 Sistemas formadores de imagen de hoy y del mañana *Electromédica* **2** 64–7

[12] Haendle J, Hohmann D and Maass W 1981 La imagen radiológica electrónica en el radiodiagnóstico preoperatorio *Electromedica* **2** 74–9

[13] Becker R 1970 Radiocinematografía con el intensificador electrónico y corriente pulsátil en el tubo *Rev. SRW* **1** 8–12

[14] General Electric Medical Systems 1987 Image enhancement primer *Product Data* 7076

[15] Bischoff K 1969 ¿La radiación pulsante tiene todavía alguna importancia en el procedimiento moderno de radiocinematografía? *Rev. SRW* **2** 56–9

[16] Reisman B 1979 The intraoperative use of the x-ray television chain with video recorder *Electromedica* **1** 15–7

[17] Batki L 1973 New image intensifier *Medicor News* **2** 19–26

[18] Udvari P 1973 Clinical experiences with the internal medical x-ray image intensifier *Medicor News* **2** 16–8

[19] Briggs E R, González Martin A and Haufe G 1983 Puesto de trabajo angiográfico universal para todas las exploraciones especiales *Electromédica* **3** 92–6

IOP Publishing

Technical Fundamentals of Radiology and CT

Guillermo Avendaño Cervantes

Chapter 11

Servo control

11.1 Introduction

One of the most effective applications of electronics is the ability to automatically maintain a stable system [1], obviously within certain limits, and electromechanical systems can be constructed which have various applications in the field of x-ray devices. The fundamental idea is servo control. Its function is to maintain an electronic circuit at a set value or in the vicinity of it, through a constant comparison between a reference value and the instantaneous value of the magnitude to be stabilized [2]. In this way some important parameters of x-ray devices can be controlled by the circuits of the device itself.

Practical applications of these systems are found in many features, for example:
- The automatic regulation of constant supply voltages.
- The automatic adjustment of alternating voltage input from the network.
- Maintaining the constant high voltage selected.
- Displaying automatic gain amplifier video on a TV system.
- The automatic adjustment of the focus–film distance (FFD) of a tube.
- The automatic adjustment of the different formats of a spot film device.
- Speed control of a tomography system.
- Automated dose adjustment through feedback timers.
- The automatic adjustment of the opening of a collimator.

As shown by these examples, there are many useful applications of these systems in practical circuits in radiology equipment. The task in some cases is to prevent a disruptive function that could affect or vary a preset value, as in the case of voltage regulators. These are circuits designed to compensate for changes in voltage, either below or above the specified value. In other cases the idea is that the servo system adjusts to different values that are selected under direct command or automatically searches for a suitable value according to some indirect requirement; as in the case of systems of automatic dose adjustment.

doi:10.1088/978-0-7503-1212-7ch11

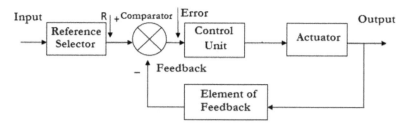

Figure 11.1. A basic servo control system.

A servo system comprises the following components:
- A controlled variable searching for the best adjustment.
- A reference value that is used for comparison.
- A comparator element that provides an output proportional to the difference between the control variable and the reference output.
- An adjustment element that changes the desired function according to the difference output from the comparator.

In practice these components have a more or less complex embodiment, according to the specific task for which the servo is utilized. In all cases the operating sequence is as follows:
1. Measure the value of the control variable.
2. Compare this to the value obtained with the reference.
3. Amplify the difference obtained by the comparator.
4. Generate a correction function.
5. Apply the correction function in a way that tends to nullify the difference obtained by the comparator.
6. Cancel the operation when it has reached the minimum difference, that is, when it has matched the reference magnitude with the regulation.

The block diagram of figure 11.1 shows a basic servo system. The sensor for measuring the desired function is a determining factor in all closed systems [3]. The comparator reference value and the control amplifier both provide the signal which acts on the adjusting element which, through the regulatory element, compensates for elements that disrupt the balance.

11.2 Power supply controller

In the case of a continuous power supply voltage, used as a simple example of such servo control functions, we need to maintain constant tension despite load variations. In this case a load change (a decrease of consumer resistance) causes an increase of the current that the power supply must deliver. This means that the voltage at the output terminals drops to values that may not be acceptable for the circuits that said power supply is feeding. The servo system should then be able to change its status so that the power supply delivers a higher current to meet the demand without changing the voltage.

Technical Fundamentals of Radiology and CT

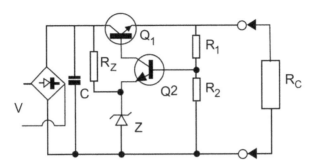

Figure 11.2. A power supply regulator circuit.

Figure 11.2 shows a power supply regulator circuit. Detecting changes in the output voltage is performed by changing the voltage across the resistor R1 by altering the voltage applied between R1 + R2. A change corresponding to each resistor divider occurs. This change voltage is measured by the comparison transistor in its base because this has a fixed voltage reference held by the Zener regulator issuer. Thus there is a voltage difference between the base and the emitter of the transistor which changes the polarization, causing it to conduct more and thus a higher voltage is applied to the transistor Q1 (connected in series). This creates variable resistance, making Q1 conduct more and thus deliver greater power. This produces the desired effect of increasing the supply voltage by providing more current. Obviously, the process described is valid within a certain level of voltage modification; for very high changes the system will be unable to correct the deviation. The opposite effect of increased tension is handled in the same vein, leading to reduced conduction of the comparison transistor Q2 and consequently reducing the conduction of the adjustment in element Q1, causing a decrease in the output current to compensate the increase.

In figure 11.3 we can see how different elements of setting, magnitudes of adjustment and magnitudes of control in a servo system are used [4]. Among the elements of a complete control system, the regulators and comparators are fundamental. Other components, such as the reference source, the sensors and the setting items, are relatively well known and conventional. Modern electronics use operational integrated circuits as comparators, some of which have a specific design for the function for which they are intended. These are relatively easy to find in any book of electronic components. For that reason, we will not explain their operation in detail.

11.3 Types of regulators

Due to the importance of regulators in radiological circuits, we will describe their classification and basic characteristics.

Regulators can be of the following types:
- Function YES–NO (ON–OFF).
- Proportional function (type P).
- Integral function (type I).

Adjust magnitude	Adjusting element	Adjustment effect	Control magnitude
Number of turns	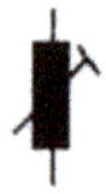 Adjustable transformer	On the transformation ratio	Voltage
Resistance considered	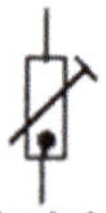 Adjustable resistor	On the voltage divider ratio	Voltage
Grid polarization	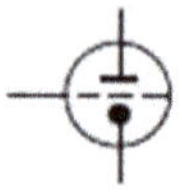 Electronic valve	On the anode current	Anode current
Base current	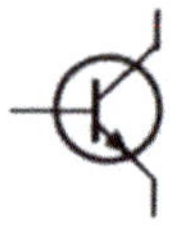 Transistor	on the collector current	collector current
Instant ignition	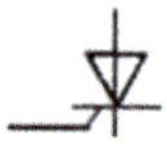 Thyristor	On the conduction angle	Anode current
Excitation current	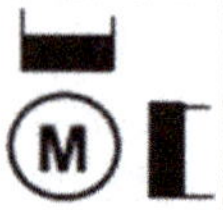 Servomotor	On the torque	Rotational movement

Figure 11.3. Factors of a servo system.

- Differential function (type D).
- Proportional differential function (PD type).
- Proportional integral differential function (PID).

The simplest regulator is called a YES–NO regulator, a function of the presence or absence of action, such as connecting a switch. This type of control is used, for example, in thermal systems. A heating circuit is fed and when the sensor detects the selected temperature level the order is sent to interrupt the current, which causes a gradual temperature drop to a lower limit, which commands reconnecting the power to seek an increase. This control string seeks to maintain

Technical Fundamentals of Radiology and CT

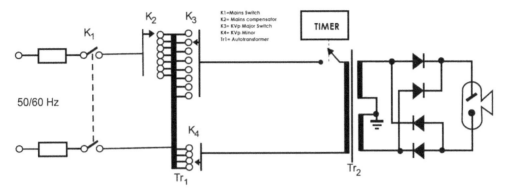

Figure 11.4. Manual adjustment of power voltage and kVp.

the temperature at a value close to the stabilization level. This type of regulator is used when the thermal inertia is high, i.e. the temperature does not drop quickly to a minimum when the current is interrupted, nor does it increases rapidly when energized by the heater circuit. This level of control is not acceptable for applications requiring greater accuracy. This is why regulators with the best characteristics are used.

The proportional controller delivers an output signal that is proportional to the input, i.e. following its behavior to the exciter function. This allows its application in systems in which a large degree of variation is required. The response is quick but has the disadvantage that its amplifications can result in oscillations, because in some cases increased gain is required to reduce the difference between the reference values and the actual values. The integral, differential and combined regulators allow us ample opportunity to apply fine-grain, fast and highly accurate regulation for all desired applications.

In radiological circuits there are, apart from the voltage regulators of many sources of power supply, systems for servo automatic setting, kVp adjustment, video control, automatic collimation and so on.

11.4 Servo adjustment of voltage power

In the devices initially described in this chapter, there is a simple and direct way to compensate for fluctuations in the supply network. If these fluctuations are not nullified they provoke an unacceptable change in the device parameters. A manual selector can be used that adjusts the connection up or down in the taps of the autotransformer input in order to offset the changes (see figure 11.4). An instrument connected to the network of the generator used permanently measures the voltage and thus the operator can visually check whether there were changes and proceed with the respective adjustments [5].

An automated adjustment system has the advantage of not requiring monitoring or operator action to make changes. An electronic circuit is responsible for continuously detecting the voltage and commands a motor to move up or down the sliding selector contact to compensate the misalignment. Motor movement ceases when the balance has been achieved, i.e. when the comparator has applied to

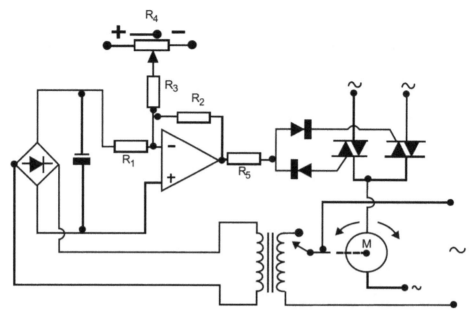

Figure 11.5. Servo adjustment of power voltage.

the equipment the exact voltage required despite changes in the supply voltage, as shown in figure 11.5.

The circuit operates as follows. While using the output value of input autotransformer, the circuit takes this voltage to the comparator in reduced form by a voltage divider to the input of an electronic comparator. The other input of the comparator is a voltage reference, such as to provide a null output to the comparator when both are equal; this output does not send any signal to the motor and it does not move.

When there is a different voltage at the input to the previous network, the input voltage changes as does the comparator output delivery, because the other input has a stabilizing voltage. Then the motor is commanded to move in the direction to compensate the misalignment by changing the adjustment slider that produces the output voltage of the autotransformer.

11.5 Servo adjustment of high voltage applied to the tube

The voltage applied to the tube should be as stable as possible, because this guarantees the possibility of repeating the selection of radiographic values, in particular the voltage, for each shot with the same results on the film. It is therefore desirable to provide circuits to maintain the fixed voltage at the selected value [6], despite the changes of supply voltage, and to stabilize the high voltage for the duration of the radiographic shot to compensate for changes caused by the load.

The simplest solution is to use manual switching contactors. In many second-generation devices they are selectable in increments of 10 kV for high values and in steps of 1 kV for small values. As the voltage can be measured instrumentally in the primary transformer, the visual appreciation of this voltage allows the operator to

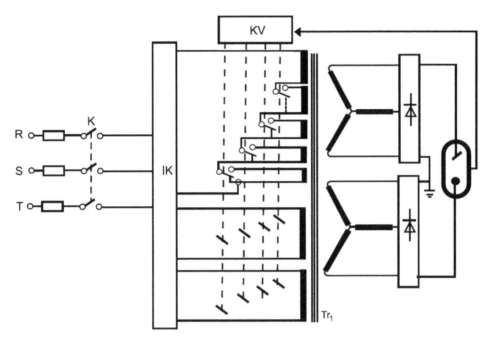

Figure 11.6. The automatic adjustment of voltage.

make corrections before the next shot if changes were made. This method is of course limited and does not allow automatic adjustment during shooting. Therefore, automated adjustment systems are designed to work at the primary side of the high voltage transformer (see figure 11.6), particularly for the fluoroscopic applications which have a duration that enables a permanent setting.

The central idea of the method is to change the connection of the coils in the primary transformer to the daily changes required and the tension adjusts itself in the transformer without load when more or fewer coils of the primary are connected, governed by a circuit that senses the real tension [7]. Figure 11.7 shows the set of blocks that are responsible for making the connections of coils. In figure 11.8, the circuit in detail is shown. The basic system operation is as follows. Through block 6 a reference network is taken and thus is controlled by the constant current generator, 8, which delivers a current value of I. This latter will generate a variable current I_0, depending on the number of leads connected in parallel to R0 through the switching transistors which are inserted from R1 to R7. That is, if all transistors are driving, all resistances are connected in parallel and current I_0 will have the smallest possible value ($I_0 = I - D_1$). The opposite occurs when no transistor is conducting: the current I_0 is the highest possible value and equal to I. The resulting current I_0, is applied to an electronic comparator, 3, which will receive two pieces of information for comparison: the I_0 values of current and another current generated in the voltage setting of tube 4, which is proportional to the kVp that the operator selects. Thus the comparator will provide a voltage which commands the control circuit, 5, driving the binary counter until the latter delivers pulses that activate, more or less,

Technical Fundamentals of Radiology and CT

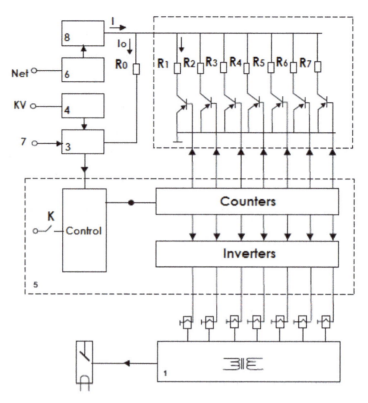

Figure 11.7. Voltage control system relays.

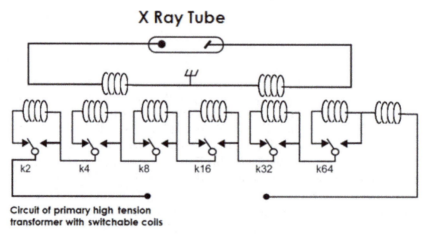

Figure 11.8. Switching of primary coils.

the switching transistors responsible for the value of the comparison current I_0. When equilibrium is reached, i.e. when the comparator output is not delivered, then the binary counter stops at a value that accurately represents the value of the selected kVp. The encoded bit value is applied simultaneously to inverters which manage the

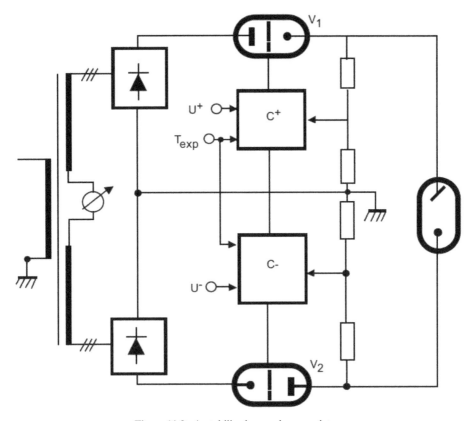

Figure 11.9. A stabilized secondary regulator.

relays in charge of connecting more or fewer coils in the high voltage transformer located in block 1.

When an abnormality of the supply voltage occurs, the value of the reference current I generated in 8 is automatically changed, and thus the value I_0, so that the comparator delivers an output which governs the counter by modifying both. The number of transistors is the same as the number of relays that are activated to connect more or fewer coils. It is understood that modifications can be increasing or decreasing in the direction of the altered line voltage.

Since switching is directed by a binary counter of seven, outputs can have a wide range of variation given by the combinatorial possibilities of seven bits, so that the automatic compensation is very broad-level and allows quick adjustment. Any other factor that causes a change of the selected voltage will create the same conditions in relation to the activity of the binary counter and adjust the values, compensating for alterations.

Changes in the current effect of the secondary load are sensed in the circuit tube and fed back through point 7 which enters in the comparator, 3. Thus there is another way of tuning over the function of the tube in situations of voltage change per load.

A final method for automated adjustment works on the transformer secondary high voltage, based on the principle of regulation of the stabilized dc voltage power supply (see figure 11.9) [8]. In this case a control circuit based on triode power is

Technical Fundamentals of Radiology and CT

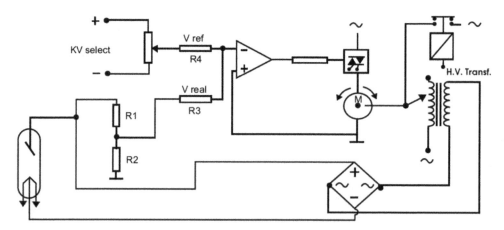

Figure 11.10. Regulation by a motorized actuator at low-level voltage comparators.

applied to both electrodes of the x-ray tube, the anode and the cathode. The triodes are connected as steps of regulation in series, using in addition a voltage divider. Applying a correction voltage to regulator block C+ or C−, or both simultaneously, the block receives a voltage governing the triode grid by driving it more or less in the direction of maladjustment compensation.

The circuit described has the advantages of being free of mechanical inertia and giving a very rapid response to the correction during the radiation. However, it is inconvenient to handle and has expensive components which require additional generation of x-rays by the tube regulators, because these are subjected to high voltages. The latter issue can be eliminated by shielding, as utilizing this method has clear benefits.

Another compensation system operates through a divider circuit that takes a sample of the circulating current of the tube (which being high produces a loading effect altering the voltage, see figure 11.10). This current is applied as a comparison value on an integrated comparator while simultaneously reaching a reference value given by the voltage selected by the operator so that the comparator output is proportional to the sum of both voltages. A signal circuit then connects a control amplifier which governs the motor of the mechanical actuator on the primary of the high voltage transformer. The motor movement is fast and smooth, adjusting the voltage such that the current of the divider in kilovolts is proportional to the voltage applied, then re-adjusting the voltage in the input of the comparator.

Note that we are using a comparison system by voltage sum at the same input of the operational circuit, and that the voltages are low, allowing more accuracy and security than when handling high voltages. At the same time the value selected by the operator can be adjusted easily by means of a potentiometer at low power. The system has safety limits for the movement of the selector in the mechanical sliding contactor of the transformer, so extreme voltages are not admitted and the circuit will be disabled before component failure damages the whole circuit.

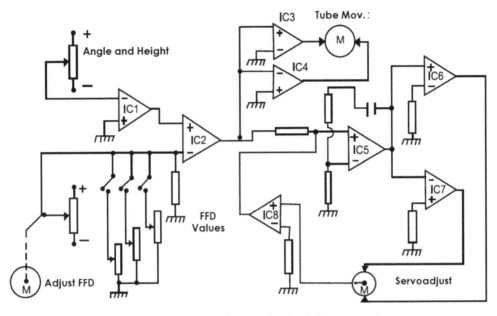

Figure 11.11. An automatic controller circuit for tomography.

11.6 Servo systems for tomography

In tomography it is necessary to automatically adjust the travel speed and direction, and correct the FFD, the cutting angle and height of the tomography slice; factors that determine the expected x-ray results. The motorized systems used have various types of sensors that feed back information instantaneously, so that the corrector setting alteration occurs in any of the parameters, as shown in figure 11.11.

In tomography this automation is more complex because not only does the actual value of a position (with error or not) need to be compared with the desired value, but also the reference values from other variables which act simultaneously in the comparison. For example, when the signal from the desired angle value and the value of the cutting height are chosen, they simultaneously determine a correction value for the speed of the tomography motor's back and forth motion, while also being necessary to correct the same movement with the signals from the FFD. This is the signal of the actual position of the tomographic mechanical bar and all possible signals from fixed values of pre-selectable FFDs (one at a time).

The outputs of the first comparator give a voltage proportional to all the factors involved, and may be positive or negative, accordingly making the correction in the direction of the disturbance compensator [9]. In turn, the value obtained is compared to another circuit with a signal from a tachometer (voltage as a function of rpm), so that this information is applied to the motor in a negative or positive sense by inverters in order to adjust the speed of the cutting angle.

11.7 Servo-adjustment of spot film devices

A spot film device should insert the cassette and place it so that it can perform the subdivision and then move away from the radiation beam. The operations that

Technical Fundamentals of Radiology and CT

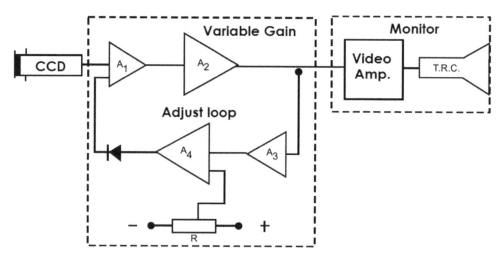

Figure 11.12. An automatic control circuit for a video image.

determine the aperture setting of the sheets that prevent full-film exposure with the first shot and the automatic opening of the collimator to the chosen format are simultaneous operations that require precise adjustment. The light beam collimator, the opening diagrams and the positioning of the cassette must be accurate for proper use of the film and to prevent information loss occurring from overlapping or cutting the radiation field.

All this is achieved through an automated adjustment using sensor, amplifier and motor regulation through feedback, permanently adjusting and accurately correcting all positions and dimensions defined by the manufacturer for each type of format and subdivision. The system is simple to describe, in particular if the operation of similar systems is understood.

A comparator receives the corresponding information from any variable's (cassette size, location, subdivision sequence) preset values. These signals can be defined by the resistance of a potentiometer which varies by a transmitter belt system dependent on an adjustable frame in which the cassette with film is installed, so that each size means a different position of the potentiometer shaft. A set of reed relays set to open or close depending on the size of the cassette can also be used.

On the other hand, the comparator receives information from a variable voltage based on the actual position of the servomotor. This is usually implemented with a potentiometer of the simultaneous movement with the motor shaft (using gears or pulley systems). If the comparator receives different signals at its output there is a voltage that is introduced to a control amplifier, which connects to a relay activation of the motor rotation direction, depending on the polarity of the comparator output, with the instruction to mobilize the motor in the search for balance. When this is achieved, the motor receives no signal and stops. This is where it will have the final positioning which must correspond to the desired size or magnitude.

All systems similar to that described have electronics and mechanical components such as gears, motors, belts, clamps and fasteners of various kinds. All can produce mismatches through use, wear and lubrication failure, producing situations of malfunction or damage that can be avoided by a policy of proper maintenance

11.8 Servo systems for video control

Any system of radiological TV images contains among its main components a closed loop automatic gain adjustment of the video. The purpose of these circuits is to maintain the output to the monitor with a constant video amplitude level, despite changes in input amplitude from the movie camera. Notable changes that occur in the magnitude of brightness due to differences in tissue density produce significant leaps in the video magnitude which need to be compensated instantly through electronic means without intervention of inertial mechanical elements.

The image signal from the camera reaches the central of the video where it is applied to a video amplifier, which takes a sample to be used in the magnitude comparison as the actual value, see figure 11.12. This is entered into the electronic comparator, which also receives a reference value determined by a potentiometer which is adjusted to the desired value. The comparator outputs a signal which is rectified and becomes a variable value of bias in the control amplifier, which in turn alters the input signal to the video amplifier compensating for changes in signal magnitude [10]. Thus the composite video signal reaches the monitor with a constant amplitude despite containing information on the full range of possible shades of gray.

References

[1] RCA Institute 1980 Electronic for automation *Training Course*
[2] Zbar P B 1997 *Industrial Electronics* (New York: McGraw-Hill)
[3] Siemens 1987 Cadenas de control y circuitos de regulación *Informationen für Med-Techniker*
[4] Davis S A and Ledgerwood B 1981 *Electromechanical Components for Servomechanisms* (New York: McGraw-Hill)
[5] Davis S 1997 *Retroalimentación y Sistemas de Control* (Mexico City: Fondo Educativo Interamericano S A)
[6] Marton A 1968 EDR 750, x-ray equipment based on a new control principle *Medicor News* **3** 51–60
[7] Siemens 1987 Etapas de pasos simatic *Informationen für Med-techniker*
[8] Aguado A and Enriquez J 1989 *Teoría Moderna de Control* (Havana: Editorial Academia)
[9] Doebelin E 1999 *Dynamic Analysis Feedback Control* (New York: McGraw-Hill)
[10] Czine J and Csontos P 1977 The necessity of frequency transformation of high speed systems regulated under exposure *Medicor News* **1** 1–8

IOP Publishing

Technical Fundamentals of Radiology and CT

Guillermo Avendaño Cervantes

Chapter 12

High frequency technique (multipulse)

12.1 Introduction

For many years, x-ray generation was based on the use of high voltages created from the network frequency, which is 50 Hz or 60 Hz. This concept requires a lot of iron in the transformer core in order to obtain high power. According to the equations used for manufacturing transformers, we obtain that the voltage induced in the transformer secondary depends on several technical factors [1]: the input voltage, the magnetic permeability of the core and the number of turns of wire used ($V_1 = 4$, $N_I = 44, f_1, \varphi_{max}$). Thus when it is necessary to have a high voltage and a high output current, many turns of wire must be used (N_I) with adequate wire gage to handle high currents. This means having enough space in the core geometry for all the wire to fit inside if the system works with a constant low frequency f_1 (50 Hz or 60 Hz).

Now if we consider that the induced voltage depends on the frequency [2], we can have the same voltage with fewer turns of wire if we increase the frequency instead of the number of turns and at the same time if a core of high permeability material is used (superior to iron) for greater magnetic flux (φ_{max}), whereby equivalent power transformers with a much smaller volume and weight are achieved. In the situation described, requiring the creation of a high frequency potential at high power [3] which is not possible with only a conventional oscillator, a system with high frequency oscillation with high power is required as is the possibility to change the output voltage for the range of voltages required for radiographs (between 40 kV and 150 kV).

As explained it is theoretically possible to obtain a high induced voltage if we have a transformer core of high magnetic permeability with an alternating high frequency voltage generated by a variable oscillator that is capable of generating high power. These voltages can be applied to the primary of the transformer, equivalent to those used in conventional x-ray technology, i.e. applying voltages of hundreds of volts to induce thousands of volts in the transformer secondary. In practical terms, the situation is not as straightforward, as in the conventional system

doi:10.1088/978-0-7503-1212-7ch12　　　　12-1　　　　© IOP Publishing Ltd 2016

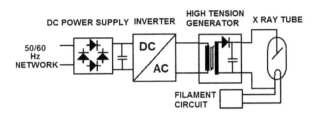

Figure 12.1. A high frequency x-ray generation system. Modified from Electromedica/Siemens.

the voltage intended to be applied on the high voltage transformer, an input autotransformer connected to the conventional electricity network, provides all the power required, which is obtained through its electrical parameters and large physical dimensions from the available mains frequency (50 Hz or 60 Hz). High frequency systems must be designed and constructed with a generator of medium voltages (hundreds of volts), which delivers high voltages (between 40 kV and 150 kV), varying the frequency (in the range of 20–40 kHz), instead of varying the input voltage as a conventional system does.

To generate x-rays with a high voltage at a different frequencies, is necessary to have a system to convert the frequency to an alternating voltage [4], then increase this tension, if possible rectifying and eventually filtering to apply this high voltage on the x-ray tube as constantly as possible.

It should be remembered that in conventional x-ray technology a very high voltage is generated from the 50 Hz or 60 Hz, which can only be rectified with devices that sustain this high voltage, but it cannot be filtered because that would require capacitors with very high voltage and high capacity, which are not commercially available. This marks a major advantage of the technique of high frequency (or multipulse), because it is possible to filter a high frequency and high voltage with capacitors that have a high dielectric strength to withstand high voltage and not a very large capacitance. Figure 12.1 shows a conceptual diagram of the generation of x-rays using a high frequency system.

12.2 How to obtain a high voltage variable frequency

The technical effort to make an oscillator system (inverter) change its frequency so as to achieve the required secondary voltages is too demanding. The solution to the problem was made possible by the existence of solid-state devices that handle high powers as in the case of controlled thyristors (silicon-controlled rectifiers (SCRs)). The circuit shown in figure 12.2 is the conceptual basis for high voltage generating systems for the so-called multipulse technique or medium frequencies. Its basis is as follows.

An RLC circuit supplied with a dc voltage generates an oscillating signal that is damped when a switch is closed. The first part of the circulating current is almost a half-sine which dampens over time, which in figure 12.2 is used as a switch to a thyristor (SCR). On receipt of the appropriate gate voltage this is brought into full conduction. Then the circuit generates a current pulse applied to the resistance which generates a half-sine form voltage.

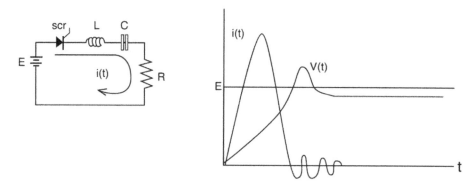

Figure 12.2. The basic circuit of damped wave generation.

We can see that the waveform of the current in its first part corresponds to a half-sine, so that if this current is applied to the primary of a transformer producing a voltage induced in the secondary with the same waveform, the system requires a complete cycle with a second half-sine but with the opposite direction, i.e. with a negative value. If this is a circuit that alternately generates these half-sines, we have a suitable waveform and the voltage required depends on the number of laps in the secondary.

The frequency at which the electronic switch (SCR) is closed determines the oscillation frequency that is generated [5]. Therefore, it is necessary to have a trigger circuit of the gates of the thyristors with the possibility of varying the frequency of pulse emission, and obviously a suitable combination of components that allows the generation of the pulses comprising the sequential damped high frequency wave oscillating circuit to alternate. The circuit shown in figure 12.3 is a conceptual diagram of this process [6].

Both triggers 1 and 3 generate positive sign waves, and triggers 2 and 4 generate negative waves. The sequence is shown on the right of the figure and gives rise to the current $i(p)$, with a sinusoidal shape to result in a current in the same way and frequency in the secondary but with a much higher voltage level.

The electronic implementation of these circuits is shown in figure 12.4, in which the thyristors are triggered in sequence so that the current follows a path that involves developing a voltage on both sides of the primary in the transformer of high frequency. Initially two thyristors opposite each other in the first bridge are shorted and current flows are damped by the upper primary of the transformer. The dashed line shows the path of the wave when it is in the first half cycle of the damped wave where the transformer alternately looks like a sine wave [7]. The resulting waveforms are shown in figure 12.5 with the pulse sequence.

12.3 A complete multipulse circuit

The initial system of x-ray generation by a high frequency ac, called 'multipulse', was created by Siemens with a conceptual scheme as shown in figure 12.6. In this block diagram we have a part of the network which feeds the three-phase converter which supplies both systems. The high frequency voltage for the anode circuit on

Technical Fundamentals of Radiology and CT

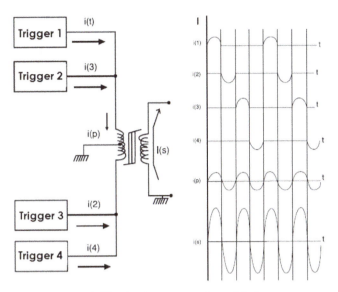

Figure 12.3. The circuit generator of a multipulse wave.

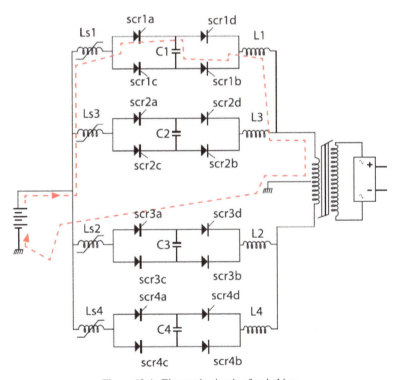

Figure 12.4. Electronic circuit of switching.

Technical Fundamentals of Radiology and CT

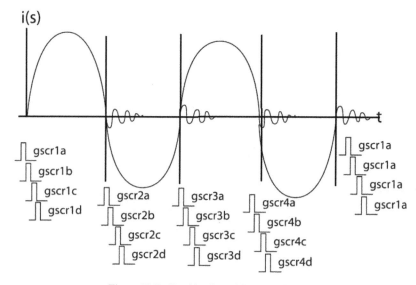

Figure 12.5. Combined resulting waveforms.

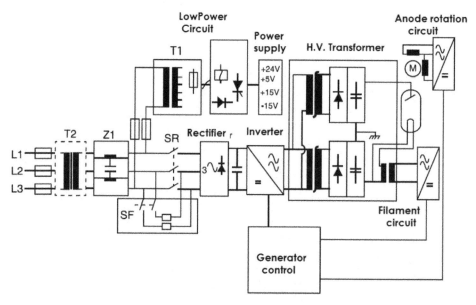

Figure 12.6. A complete multipulse generation system. Modified from Electromedica/Siemens.

the tube and the tube filament power supply circuit are provided through high frequency transformers and their respective rectifying and filtering circuits [8]. This stage has the option of applying tension in fluoroscopy or radiography. At the same time the power is supplied to the conventional low voltage source intended for electronics and the connection to the central control with which the current values, voltage and duration of the radiographic shot are selected, and finally the rotation control circuit, a condition necessary to authorize emission of x-rays.

References

[1] General Electric Medical Systems 1989 X-ray generators *Training Course*

[2] Seibert J A 1997 The AAPM/RSNA physics tutorial for residents: x-ray generators *RadioGraphics* **17** 1533

[3] Siemens 1987 Componentes analógicos digitales de los generadores MP *Informationen für Med-Techniker*

[4] Krestel E 1990 *Imaging Systems for Medical Diagnostics* (New York: Wiley)

[5] Penketh J R 1982 *Electronic Power Control for Technicians* (Butterworths Technician Series) (Oxford: Butterworth-Heinemann)

[6] Breitling G and Noske Y E 1981 Polyphos 300, un generador radiológico de frecuencia media *Electromédica* **2** 113–21

[7] Hino H, Hatakeyama T, Kawase T and Nakaoka M 1989 High-frequency parallel resonant converter for x-ray generator utilizing parasitic circuit constants of high voltage transformer and cables *Proc. 11th Int. Telecommunications Energy Conf. (15–18 Oct 1989, Florence, Italy)* vol 2 (Piscataway, NJ: IEEE) p 20.5/1

[8] Sobol W T 2002 High frequency x-ray generator basics *Med. Phys.* **2** 132–44

IOP Publishing

Technical Fundamentals of Radiology and CT

Guillermo Avendaño Cervantes

Chapter 13

CT principles and fundamentals

13.1 Introduction

Although the resulting images from CT studies are analyzed by a radiologist in the same way as the x-ray films obtained by any of the conventional radiographic methods, it can be categorically stated from the technical point of view that CT marks a true revolution in the field of radiology [1]. It is the first technology introduced since the invention of the first x-ray device that is successfully able to compete with traditional x-ray devices. This reflects the fact that no significant advances were achieved in producing radiographic images from 1895 until 1972, when CT was introduced, despite the optimization of tubes and screens, the introduction of image intensification and radiological TV, and a series of improvements in the components of radiological systems. The importance of CT has been recognized by the international scientific community, who granted its inventor, the English scientist C R Hounsfield, the 1979 Nobel Prize in medicine. The unit for determining the scale of the absorption coefficients is known as the Hounsfield unit (HU) [2].

Before CT, the only method for obtaining valid images for diagnosis was to make x-rays pass through the body of the patient and collect the dimmed beam of x-rays reflecting the different densities of the components of the body on a photographic film. This classical method [3], which of course will continue to be used for the foreseeable future, involves two major disadvantages. In traditional x-rays, information from three dimensions is overlapped on a single plane, which can make diagnosis difficult. Also, the organic components that present great variation in their absorption of x-rays in relation to neighboring tissues produce enough contrast so that the eye of the radiologist can distinguish them, but among tissues with similar absorption of radiation it is not possible to differentiate between structures. The practical drawbacks of both these disadvantages can be appreciated from figures 13.1 and 13.2.

Due to these drawbacks x-ray images of organs located in the brain cavity could not be obtained, apart from films obtained of the ventricles after the introduction of

doi:10.1088/978-0-7503-1212-7ch13   13-1   © IOP Publishing Ltd 2016

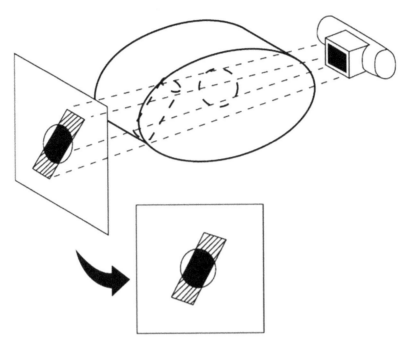

Figure 13.1. A conventional image with superimposed structures.

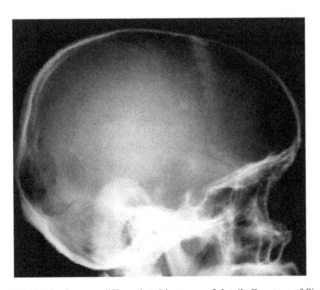

Figure 13.2. Brain tissue undifferentiated in terms of detail. Courtesy of Siemens.

air or a mixture of iodine for visualization of brain vessels, in procedures invented by Dandy and Moniz, respectively [4]. It was impossible to differentiate anything else within the skull.

In an attempt to overcome this important limitation, various scientists tried procedures designed to obtain further information, in particular on brain and vessel tissue. However, all these techniques have various disadvantages, in particular the necessity for hospitalization, the risk of injury or damage, and the need for highly qualified staff [5]. Also, several of these procedures produce a high irradiation for the patient and staff.

For these reasons, it was necessary to develop a procedure that would eliminate or compensate for the disadvantages of conventional x-rays, in particular for studies of the cranial cavity. Thus a technique was designed to obtain images that might be equivalent to the tomographic procedures already discussed, with the notable difference that the radiation should be screened, not along the surface as in planigraphic studies, but around the skull, with the emitter rotating around the head. This original idea is the basis of the conception of the current CT technique and explains the term 'axial' in computed axial tomography.

Conventional axial x-ray tomography has been used for many years to obtain radiographs of the maxillofacial region, including cervical tomograms, with a number of advantages over other procedures [6], which are valid only in the study of bone, joints and teeth. However, there still remained the problem that both sides of the skull produced images without any useful information from the inside, therefore, it was necessary to devise a procedure that allowed a quantitative assessment of the radiation absorption ability of different tissues within the cranial cavity.

13.2 A historical summary of CT

Over the decades, researchers worked towards designing a method of using radiation that would display on a graphic document (the film), the differences in tissue densities of the head. As part of this effort devices and procedures were invented that did not go beyond the traditional framework of x-ray emission, the interposition of the object and the impression on a film. Therefore, significant results were not obtained until the topic was considered in terms of the radiation absorbed by biological tissue profiles. The central idea in this concept was the correct assumption that different types of tissue would present different absorption of x-rays, which should be reflected in some mathematical way.

The aim was to achieve something already known in the physical sciences, the reconstruction of the structure of internal objects by means of its projections. This method was well known in the exact sciences and biology, for example: applications in cytology for the reconstruction of very small cells with very complex structures; the determination of regions of the Sun that emit microwaves; and its use in radio astronomy and electron microscopy. Therefore, the attempt of the inventors of CT was preceded by a solid and reliable history of implementing procedures for two-dimensional or three-dimensional reconstruction in scientific research.

The first step was made by a German mathematician at the beginning of the twentieth century, J Radon, who published in Leipzig in 1917, an article which outlined the basis for the mathematical procedure that would be later used for the above-mentioned scientific applications [7]. Among these applications was the study carried out in 1956 by R N Bracewell, who used microwave radiation measurements from Sun in different projections [8]. That is, he was able to measure the total radiation in each direction then reconstruct a two-dimensional map through using the equations and mathematical methods introduced by Radon. Studies on bio-medical applications carried out at the beginning of the 1960s by three different groups of unrelated researchers (those of Kuhl (radio-isotope) from University of Pennsylvania, Bracewell (radio-astronomy) from Stanford University and Oldendorf (physiology) from UCLA California) were taken into account by the creators of CT as background precursors to develop their fundamental idea.

In 1961 W Oldendorf used a method called spin migration to rebuild the profiles of radiation absorption in a block of plastic with small pieces of iron and aluminum inserted in it [9]. The experiment consisted of the irradiation of a $10 \times 10 \ cm^2$ block of plastic using a collimated source of gamma rays. The block was placed on a turntable plate turning at a velocity of 16 rpm, with its center of rotation being simultaneously shifted in a linear fashion at a rate of 8 cm h^{-1} by a clockwork mechanism. The radiation transmitted through the object was collected by a solid-state detector (NaI) associated with a photomultiplier tube. From there it was sent to an electronic circuit designed to filter and graphically record the different projections.

The main idea was to produce modulation of the beam by the linear movement of the metal chips embedded in the block. Since the linear movement was slower than the rotational speed, the low pass filter could separate the two frequencies and preserve only the effect of the linear movement on the beam. The process had the disadvantage of extending the reconstruction time. The consequent increase of the radiation dose make this method inappropriate for practical applications on living tissue. However, the reconstruction results were conclusive in terms of the possibility of obtaining certain determinations of radiation absorption within an object.

In 1963, Kuhl and Edwards published an article in the journal *Radiology*, which described the procedure of reconstruction of tomographic images using radio-isotopes [10]. These images were reconstructed using simple methods of back projection, which are valid procedures in general, but which have very little determinative or diagnostic value. Certainly a more elaborate mathematical method of reconstruction and the eventual use of computers in modern devices would yield more informative images. However, the problem of exposure to high levels of radiation due to long scan times remained a serious obstacle.

The first researcher to apply a procedure of reconstruction with the use of x-rays was the physicist A Cormack, of Tufts University. He developed a mathematical method of calculation for the distribution of x-ray absorption from the values being explored with radiation [11]. He was also the first scientist who had knowledge of the Radon publications and used them as a basis for applications in medicine. Cormack embraced the idea of the measurement of the transmission of x-rays along parallel lines in a large number of different directions to obtain a sequence of profiles of x-ray transmission. These multiple profiles can be subjected to Fourier analysis to reconstruct the coefficients of linear absorption (G), whose polar coordinates would be (r, Φ) of the area being explored.

Cormack carried out experiments using a source of gamma radiation with a re-collimated beam with a width of 7 mm, and measured the intensity of the transverse beam with a 5 min interval using a Geiger–Müller counter. A cylinder surrounded by a ring of wood was studied and the absorption coefficients were calculated. Cormack then realized that his results were applicable in the field of radiology, since an x-ray beam could replace the source used in their experiment for the determination of absorption coefficient variables in two dimensions. The theoretical conception of Cormack contains the essence of CT and resulted in his sharing the Nobel Prize with G Hounsfield, the renowned inventor of CT.

Between the work by Cormack described above and the year 1967, when Hounsfield began his work in the central laboratory for research of the British electronics company EMI, some studies were carried out that came to complement the theoretical and experimental basis on which the first device useable with patients was developed in 1971. Some of the studies that should be mentioned include those by Tretiak, Eden, Simon [12] and the team of Bates and Peters. The first oral reports about the invention of CT and its applications were made in 1972 and the first articles were published in 1973 by G Hounsfield and his medical collaborator J Ambrose.

The initial prototype head scanner was installed in 1971 at Atkinson Morley's Hospital, London, UK; 2011 was the 40th anniversary of the commercial use of CT technology. Simultaneously, EMI began manufacturing the device at a larger scale, with its first model, generically referred to as 'Scanner', appearing on the market in 1973. EMI supplied a total of 60 systems around the world by 1974, with the notable distinction of being a company totally unrelated to the field of radiology. This was one of the reasons for EMI abandoning the manufacture of such devices some years later.

The initial success of EMI was a shock for companies with an emphasis on radiological work. Many executives wondered why they themselves had not been forerunners of this new and revolutionary technology, which was also very promising from the point of view of demand. Many radiologists and physicians requested such devices, and most significant medical centers considered the CT scanner to be a key piece of equipment, a matter of the highest priority. The projections made in terms of demand were valid, and the data collected show that in the first ten years [13] after their introduction into medical practice, the number of CT scanners in use rose to 7000 (see figure 13.3).

The rapid development of CT caused, in a few years, remarkable improvements which have led to devices with the current levels of high sophistication and innovation [14]. Soon the full body tomograph was produced, along with dramatic reductions in scan times and important changes in the mechanisms of tube movement and the optimization of detectors, giving rise to the different generations of scanners, which are categorized by their different modes of exploring the patient and collecting information.

Initially only EMI covered the world market, then in 1974 three other companies developed devices using the same principle. Thus Artronix created the first rotation–rotation system, the Ohio Nuclear Company incorporated the original

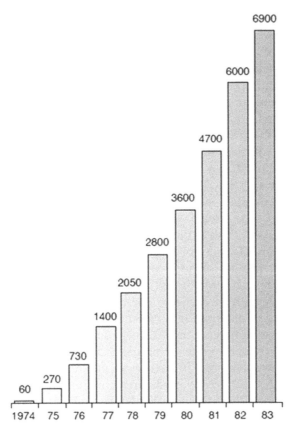

Figure 13.3. The number of CT devices installed in the first ten years after its invention. Courtesy of Siemens.

translation–rotation system and multiple detectors, and Siemens introduced the first device manufactured by a company with a tradition in radiology, the model Siretom. This preserved the rotation–translation system, which was abandoned the following year for a whole-body model and a rotation–rotation system in 1975.

In 1975, the significant producer of radiology systems, General Electric, joined in, beginning development with the rotation–rotation system, which was used for many years and was the basis of operation used by most manufacturers. That same year, Hitachi successfully covered the Japanese market with its first device for use in studies of the head. Also in 1975, Pfizer manufactured the first whole-body device (the Automatic Computerized Transverse Axial Scanner (ACTA)), which had been presented the previous year at the traditional Congress of Radiology of Chicago (RSNA), by its inventor physicist R Ledley of Georgetown University.

From that time the increase in the number of manufacturers was remarkable. Many companies saw a very promising future in this activity and in 1977 there were already 18 manufacturers, who strove to win the attention of potential customers by offering innovations and advantages in their devices. The rotation method of forming the tube into a ring with fixed detectors was invented and introduced to the market in 1976 by AS & E, and this system is still used by some manufacturers.

Later more powerful computing systems were incorporated, as well as more and better detectors. Digital x-rays were added to select the region for the tomographic cuts and improvements were also made to the following: the possibilities of image analysis; the measurements of distances; histograms, lengthening and zoom; analysis of the image for radiation therapy approaches; reconstruction of coronal and sagittal views from axial images; serial tomograms; the possibilities of studying bodies in motion, such as cardiac studies; dynamic images, etc. Subsequently, helical multislice tomography was created, which deserves a special mention for being the most powerful contemporary tool of analysis. This large universe of possibilities has made CT one of the most powerful diagnostic technologies ever invented.

In the midst of all this development, many innovations were proposed and some were adopted on a limited basis, for example, the system of movement called nutating, in which the tube turns on the outside of an inclined ring receiving radiation in one part of the detectors at a time. This system was proposed and produced in limited quantities by EMI, and was later distributed by the firm Omnimedical which did not exceed the results already known. This is why this method was not incorporated by leading firms until much later. Another system that was proposed was the ring detector with three x-ray tubes, which was assumed would lead to a significant shortening of exploration time, but this device was not successful.

In later years the commercial and technical activity in the field of CT has been restricted to six companies in Western countries [15], three in Japan (Toshiba, Hitachi and Shimatzu) and two in former Eastern-block countries (Medicor in Hungary and Tomograf in the USSR). Currently production continues to be restricted to the more powerful enterprises because only those companies have the economic capabilities for the production of this complex and expensive technology. This is largely explained by the fact that only companies that have a strong presence and enough experience in the field of radiology and biomedical equipment in general can offset the costs, invest in theoretical scientific development and compete aggressively in the market. This also explains the disappearance of some producers, who either were not able to compete or were absorbed by other, more powerful companies, as was the case for CGR and Technicare which have been acquired by General Electric. At present, there are three significant producers of CT devices in the world: Siemens, which is powerful in Europe and parts of Latin America; General Electric in the US and also in Latin America; and Toshiba, which is strong in Japan and the rest of Asia.

2011 was the 40th anniversary of the world's first clinical CT scan (1st October 1971) which was carried out at Atkinson Morley's Hospital, London, UK [16].

Most modern devices have characteristics that we will study in more detail, for example: the speed and reliability provided by computer systems, which allow shorter times for the reconstruction of images; the time of examination of the patient, which is reaching its limit due to the mechanical constraints of the system; the remarkable progress made in the quality of images, accomplished by the optimization of detectors; better algorithms and mathematical procedures for processing; and the quality of generators and tubes. High heat dissipation tubes have been developed and constructed specifically for CT. The development of powerful software packages intended for almost unlimited management of the image has also been of great importance. There are suitable image display processors to operate separate consoles that can, simultaneously with the acquisition of signals, analyze images already acquired at any time by electronically linking to the main computer. There is a global standardization aimed at the exchange of information by means of protocols such as DICOM, integrated systems for the exchange of in-hospital information with other processes such as RIS and in general HIS. Image storage capacity has increased noticeably in hard disks, magnetic tape and clouds. Finally, there is the ability to create images in three dimensions and dynamically with high resolution and image quality.

References

[1] Horn E 1978 X-ray computed tomography: medical instruments *Electron. Power* **24** 34–41

[2] Kreel L 1978 Computerized tomography using the EMI general purpose scanner *Xtract* **50** 2–14

[3] Csontos M 1978 Medicor CT, a precision neuroradiological tomodensitometer *Medicor News* 3 77–81

[4] Vallée B 1998 Subarachnoid hemorrhage syndrome and its aneurysmal etiology. From Morgagni to Moniz, Dott and Dandy. A historical overview *Neurochirurgie* **2** 5–10

[5] Kreel L 1976 The EMI whole body scanner an interim, clinical evaluation of the prototype *Br. J. Clin. Equip.* **1** 220–7

[6] Hill K R 1976 EMI total body scanner, technical aspects *Br. J. Clin. Equip.* **1** 207–14

[7] Radon J 1917 On the determination of functions from their integrals along certain manifolds *Ber. Saechsische Akad. Wiss* **29** 262

[8] Bracewell R N 1956 Strip integration in radio astronomy *Aust. J. Phys.* **9** 198–217

[9] Oldendorf W H 1961 Isolated flying spot detection of radiodensity discontinuities— displaying the internal structural pattern of a complex object *IRE Trans. Biomed. Electron.* **8** 68–72

[10] Kuhl D E and Edwards R O 1963 Image separation radioisotope scanning *Radiology* **80** 653–62

[11] Cormack A 1973 Computerized transverse axial tomography *Br. J. Radiol.* **46** 148–9

[12] Tretiak O, Eden M and Simon M 1967 *The Physical Aspects of Diagnostic Radiology* (New York: Harper)

[13] Dummling K 1984 10 años de tomografía computarizada visión retrospectiva *Electromédica* **1** 13–28

[14] Rogalsky W 1976 The Delta Sean, a unit for whole computerized tomography, technical fundamentals *Electromédica* **4** 116–23

[15] General Electric 1986 Introduction to computed tomography *General Electric Bull.*

[16] Impact Scan Org 2013 A brief history of CT http://www.impactscan.org/CThistory.htm

IOP Publishing

Technical Fundamentals of Radiology and CT

Guillermo Avendaño Cervantes

Chapter 14

On-screen CT

14.1 Introduction

In the process of obtaining a CT image with diagnostic value, a range of different factors closely related to the technology of the device are taken into account. Similarly to how the same results cannot be obtained with an amateur photography camera as with a high quality professional device, similar tomographic images cannot be obtained with early devices compared to modern systems which possess abundant improvements. Different manufacturers will take care to apply the most modern and advanced technology to achieve the ultimate priority, high quality of the image. Figure 14.1 shows the development in the quality of images on computers from the beginning of CT until today (labelled 'now' in the image). Current devices enable spectacular results and are examined in the following pages.

Obtaining images involves: acquiring the data by means of radiation applied around the object; the creation of attenuation profiles [1]; the calculation of coefficients; the assignment of values on a grayscale; and the formation of an image on the screen using these values. All of these operations will be discussed in terms of the technical significance of each step of the sequence.

14.2 In comparison to conventional radiography

Figure 14.2 shows the process of irradiating a body and the image obtained on the film in the process of obtaining a conventional radiological image. The result on the film is the depiction of a volume in a single plane, that is, we obtain a two-dimensional image of a three-dimensional object. Although the image is of high diagnostic quality, it has the drawback of overlapping structures and thus information is lost.

CT also produces two-dimensional images [2], but with the important difference that they correspond to values of radiation absorption volumes, i.e. the so-called volume elements, these are the result of an arbitrary division into numerous equal parts (cubes or volumes) of a slice of the body being scanned. This does not involve

doi:10.1088/978-0-7503-1212-7ch14   © IOP Publishing Ltd 2016

Technical Fundamentals of Radiology and CT

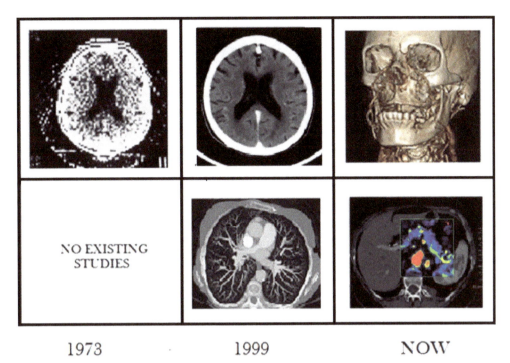

Figure 14.1. Changes in CT images over time. Courtesy of Philips.

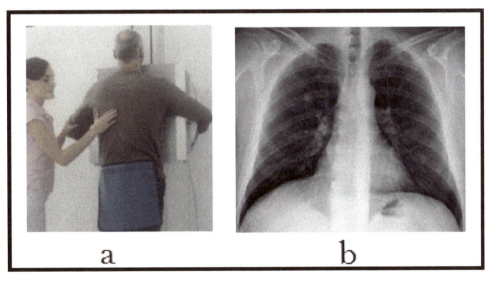

Figure 14.2. The conventional x-ray (a) process and (b) result. Courtesy of Siemens.

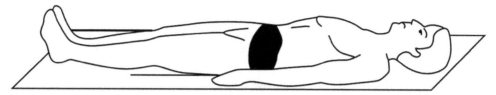

Figure 14.3. A region explored by CT.

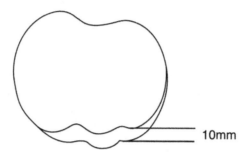

Figure 14.4. The form of an explored layer.

superimposing structures and achieves a two-dimensional image representing a nearly three-dimensional slice, as if it were a mechanical slice through that body part. The advantages of this are obviously significant and CT has revolutionized radiology [3].

Figure 14.3 shows the body region that is scanned and then displayed in the image (figure 14.4). The region has a length, width and depth, which correspond to the width of the radiation beam traversing the body. Later we will see that the beam width has a great importance in image quality, because it determines the depth of the strata explored. There are already values regulated by thickness and their importance on the image quality.

14.3 Concepts associated with the explored layer

Layers corresponding to that in figure 14.4 can be observed in any region of the patient's trunk, with an inclination to increase the beam width of the radiation applied. On the screen that shows the image obtained, only a two-dimensional plane is observed, for which we must define some important concepts [4].

14.3.1 Field of view

The magnitude of the scanned area is defined as the field of view (FOV), i.e. the entire area of the two-dimensional plane of the layer (see figure 14.5).

14.3.2 The matrix

The matrix is an array of rows and columns into which the FOV is divided (see figure 14.6). It provides an array of numbers, each one of which represents the value of the image at that location. Thus the basic purpose of the computer equipment used in CT is to calculate the numerical value assigned to each volume array, which, incidentally, corresponds to the value of the radiation absorption coefficient of each

Technical Fundamentals of Radiology and CT

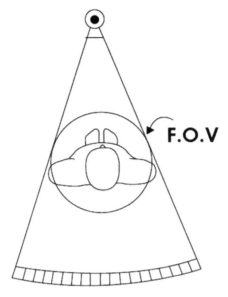

Figure 14.5. FOV.

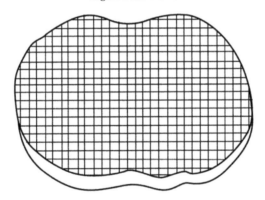

Figure 14.6. A matrix.

volume. The smaller the matrix grid separation is, the more detailed and diagnostic information will be obtained in the image, i.e. for a division of the matrix into a larger number of rows and columns. The limits to the size of the matrix are imposed by technical difficulties and cost [5].

14.3.3 The pixel

Each two-dimensional grid cell into which the FOV is divided is called a pixel (short for picture element, see figure 14.7).

14.3.4 The voxel

The volume formed by the pixel as a two-dimensional surface and the stratum width as the third dimension, is defined as the voxel (short for volume element, see figure 14.8). This is considered as the smallest volume that absorbs the applied radiation [6].

Technical Fundamentals of Radiology and CT

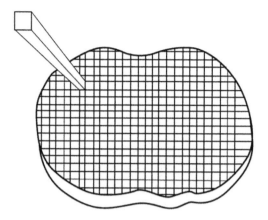

Figure 14.7. A pixel or picture element.

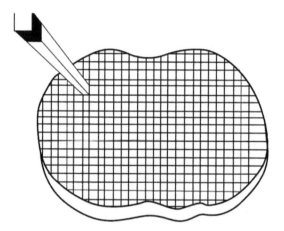

Figure 14.8. A voxel or volume element.

14.3.5 The CT number

The numerical value within a limited scale, which is assigned via previous calculations to each pixel and represents the absorption capacity of x-rays of each voxel layer or stratum studied, is defined as the CT number [7] (see figure 14.9).

14.3.6 Grayscale

For an image showing the region within the FOV, as it would look if it were the result of a physical cut through the region, a correspondence is required between the stepped tissue absorption values and staggered gray values, from intense black to absolute white (see figure 14.10). The grayscale is useful for assigning a tone of gray (or an assigned color) for each value calculated by the computer, from the different absorption coefficients scanned in the layer that correspond to each voxel. In arrays with a small number of rows and columns the points of the image appear as small squares, while for matrices with a lot of pixels we have a more harmonized image and almost cannot distinguish the small squares in the image.

Technical Fundamentals of Radiology and CT

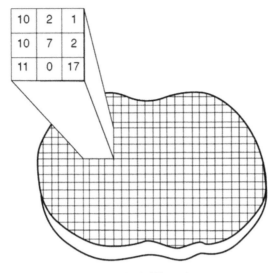

Figure 14.9. A CT number.

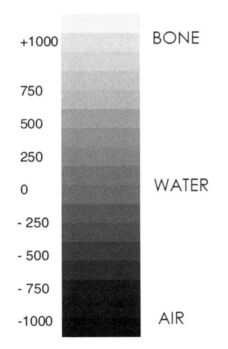

Figure 14.10. Grayscale in an image.

14.3.7 CT number scale, or Hounsfield scale

To represent the numeric values of each pixel, is necessary to use a numerical scale that quantitatively assesses the attenuation coefficient of each voxel (see figure 14.11). This scale was arbitrarily defined at the dawn of this technique with a range between +500 and –500. The maximum negative value, –500, corresponding to air,

Technical Fundamentals of Radiology and CT

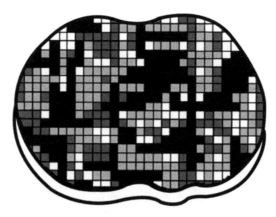

Figure 14.11. CT number scale or Hounsfield scale.

shows that it is less capable of attenuation that anything found in the body and, at the other end, the value of maximum absorption of radiation, +500, corresponds to bone. Currently, all modern systems use an extended scale of −1000 to +1000, which allows many computers to display an image with an increased scale for bone from +1000 to +3000, allowing the more in-depth study of bone disease. The middle value of the scale corresponds to the attenuation or absorption of radiation by water. Given the large number of possible values of absorption of radiation found in this scale [8], it is understandable that the human eye cannot discriminate all these values, so in obtaining image and assigning gray values the physiology of the observer must be accommodated.

14.3.8 The window

Because each gray level corresponds to an attenuation level, there are more than 2000 possible gray values represented on a monitor when an image is created from the calculated values. However, the human eye can distinguish only about 20 levels of gray, so the observer cannot obtain an adequate discrimination of differences, so a significant amount of useful information may be lost. For this reason the so-called observation window was created, the ability to expand or collapse certain regions, in order to assign different values of gray, from black to white (see figure 14.12). Thus, a narrow window displays a smaller selection of CT numbers, by which the difference can be seen between one number relative to another. Furthermore, a wide range of windows can condense several CT numbers into the same tone of gray, but can also exhibit a broad range of CT numbers.

CT devices usually have potentiometric control of the window by the operator, with a numeric display next to the image showing the limits of the window being used. Figure 14.13 illustrates the action of the control window over a range of 350. In the top panel of the sequence shown, for the value of +100 only bony areas are visible, with only the ribs and vertebrae sharply defined. In the middle panel, with a window value of 0, most thoracic tissues and muscles to the skin surface are visible [9]. Finally, in the bottom panel, with a window value of −250, the lungs filled with

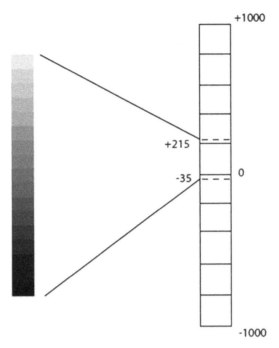

Figure 14.12. A window.

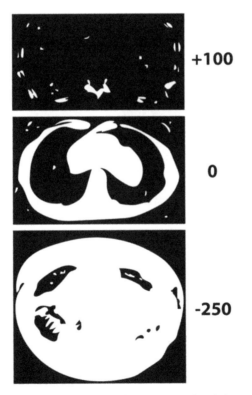

Figure 14.13. The effect of control over the window.

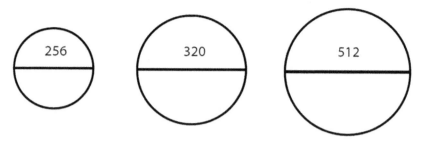

Figure 14.14. Matrix sizes.

air are visible, whereas they appeared vaguely as a black spot in the previous panel with a window of 0.

14.3.9 Relations between parameters

The most relevant concepts define some parameters that are key features of the final image. Thus the FOV, the matrix, the pixel size, the Hounsfield scale, etc, are related to each other so the technician can quantify their connections in order to define the technical performance [9].

14.3.10 Array size

The number of pixels defines the size of the array, so that different matrix values are obtained. The most widely used values in different commercial devices are 256, 320, 512 and 1024 (see figure 14.14). The dimension is defined by the number of pixels found in the horizontal or vertical image diameter.

The pixel size, as already explained, determines the image quality, and is defined as the ratio between the size of the scanned area (FOV) and the size of the array. So if we have a large matrix or a small FOV, we can obtain smaller pixel sizes which provide a greater ability to see small details, thus a better spatial resolution is achieved:

$$FOV = (pixel\ size)/(array\ size).$$

Examples of pixel size:
Example 1. FOV = 250 mm, matrix size = 256, pixel size = 1 mm.
Example 2. Minor FOV = 150 mm, matrix size = 256, pixel size ⩽ 0.6 mm.
So we obtain a better result in case 2. Note that the array size is the subdivision of the image into grid cells, according to powers of the number 2 base of the binary system: $256 = 2^8$; $512 = 2^9$; $1024 = 2^{10}$.

14.3.11 Calculation of CT numbers

The CT numbers determine the equation that relates the attenuation values of water and any biological tissue according to the scale used. Thus we have that every number becomes:

$$CT\ number = 1000 \times (\mu_{object} - \mu_{water})/\mu_{water}.$$

Water is used as the reference element for medical purposes since it is preferable not to express units in absolute terms [10], and because when the first device was made, the designer used a water bag as a compensating body, to prevent the irregular hardening of radiation while fixing the object to study.

References

[1] Siemens 1983 Fundamentos de la tomografía computarizada *Information for Medical Technicians*

[2] Fuhrer K and Liebetruth R 1975 Siretom un equipo de tomografía transversal para cráneo con computador *Electromédica* **2–3** 48–55

[3] Joubert M J 1976 Computerized axial tomography *S. Afr. Med. J.* **50** 1103

[4] General Electric Medical Systems 1986 Introduction to computed tomography *Gen. Electric Bull.* **1** 1–9

[5] Hacker H 1975 Prueba clínica del Siretom *Electromédica,* **2–3** 56–61

[6] Linke G, Pauli K and Pfeiler M 1976 Carga radiógena del paciente durante la obtención de tomografías con computadora *Electromédica* **1** 15–8

[7] Brooks R A and Dichiro G 1986 Principles of computer assisted tomography (CAT) in radiographic and radioisotopic imaging *Phys. Med. Biol.* **21** 689

[8] Siemens 1984 Fundamentos de tomografía computarizada Siretom 2000 y somatom *Information for Medical Technicians*

[9] General Electric Medical Systems 1988 CT traveler (module 1) *Sales Data*

[10] General Electric Medical Systems 1981 CT/T continum, evaluation criteria *Booklet* ICR

IOP Publishing

Technical Fundamentals of Radiology and CT

Guillermo Avendaño Cervantes

Chapter 15

Principles of CT

15.1 Introduction

The basic concept and difference of CT compared to any other method of radiological imaging is the formation of composite images for display on a computer [1] (see figure 15.1). The x-ray absorption values of different biological tissues found in the studied region are used to create the corresponding image.

To achieve this it is necessary to perform an axial scan around the object with an x-ray emitter that moves circularly. A detector system receives the amount of radiation that has managed to pass through the tissue. Since there is a direct and quantifiable relationship between the absorption of x-rays and tissue density [2], the tissues can be represented by their different densities according to their rate of absorption of radiation in an image that graphically expresses the different absorption coefficients in a bi-dimensional plane.

15.2 Density and attenuation

X-rays emitted by a tube go through the object, and when they reach the detector they only show a total attenuation of radiation in that direction (see figure 15.2). When a high number of directions is chosen, a set of total attenuations is consequently obtained. With this a set of equations can be created where the unknowns are the singular values of attenuation of each of the parts traversed by the radiation beam in that direction. Thus we can calculate the characteristic attenuation values of the small voxels into which the object under study is divided. Subsequently a shade of gray is allocated to these values, from white for the bones to black representing air, with which each specific tissue can be identified. The result on the screen of a monitor is an image built on computer-based numerical values, which appear as shades of gray [3], corresponding to an axial section of a slice of the scanned object.

doi:10.1088/978-0-7503-1212-7ch15 15-1 © IOP Publishing Ltd 2016

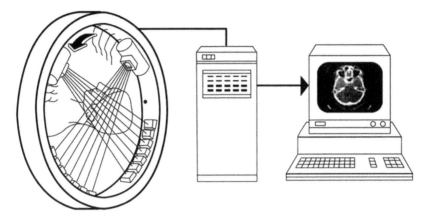

Figure 15.1. Diagram of a CT system. Courtesy of Siemens.

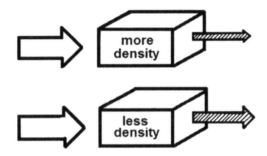

Figure 15.2. The effect of density in the transmission of x-rays.

For these reasons it follows that to study the fundamentals of CT, it is necessary to consider a number of factors that determine the quality of the resulting image:
- Absorption of radiation.
- Scanning and detection technology.
- Mathematical analysis of the detected values.
- Technical factors of image reconstruction.
- Accessories and complements to the system.

In assessing a CT system, not only do these aspects need to be taken into account, but also issues with regard to assessing dose and patient safety, as well as the safety of the personnel using the equipment [4]. The degree to which a system could be innovated with new technical developments depends on the rationality of the system and the organization of the different parts of the device in the space available.

In the acquisition of a device, it is very important to consider the degree of continuity of technical support that the manufacturer can provide, e.g. qualified personnel and spare parts, all of which are related to the size and reliability of the manufacturer. This latter is based on the experience of some companies that were unable to afford the costs of production in relation to the limited demand for devices, and which had to suspend the manufacture thereof to the detriment of users who had acquired some units. This explains the current production of CT systems being concentrated in fewer than ten powerful companies. In an article published in 1984, analyzing ten years of CT sales, K Dummling explains how some smaller companies had to leave the market in 1977 due to low demand for their devices [5].

Currently, more than 40 years after the first commercial devices were introduced, the optimization of technology has enabled price reduction and a clear improvement in the technical innovations of the different systems. Moreover, now CT has to compete with a strong rival in diagnostic imaging, nuclear magnetic resonance imaging, which in some respects exceeds the results of CT.

15.3 Absorption of radiation

The penetration into the material depends on the electrical power applied to the x-ray tube, more specifically the voltage between electrodes, according to the following formula:

$$\lambda_{min} = 12.35 \, kV^{-1}(\text{Å}).$$

The wavelength of the radiation associated with penetration is inversely proportional to the voltage applied to the tube. Therefore, the penetration of biological tissue will be ensured through a choice in the radiological generator of suitable values of voltage and the stability of the chosen values. The importance of this particular point will be emphasized later.

The value of the absorption coefficients of x-rays of different masses depends on:
– The frequency of x-ray radiation (wavelength).
– The concentration of the atomic number, i.e. the density of the absorbing x-ray material.
– The atomic number of the material in the path of the radiation beam.

For organic substances such as muscles, tendons, etc, the specific weight can be the most usual variable that is correlated with the relative absorption coefficients. Because these tissues have approximately the same proportions of carbon, nitrogen, oxygen and hydrogen, the most distinguishing feature between them is their respective density. Of course, this is not valid for special substances such as bone, which contains calcium, or for the substances of high atomic number used for contrast. These features should be considered for the proper interpretation of the values of the relative absorption coefficients. Fortunately, the importance of CT diagnosis is evident specifically in these organic substances with similar characteristics (soft tissues), which are not efficiently detected using conventional x-ray techniques.

It has been observed that the absorption coefficients relating to the biological tissues of low atomic number are related more to the electron density than the mass density. This is consistent with the theory of absorption of x-rays, which postulates the following concerning the atomic number: absorption is proportional to the cube of the atomic number with reference to hydrogen ($Z = 1$). The importance of this observation can be noted in the case of blood; a calculation shows that the difference between the electronic densities of normal and coagulated blood is not as large as the difference between their mass densities, and therefore an image obtained with CT will not reflect large difference in these types of blood.

To be able to discriminate differences between tissues with very close relative absorption coefficients [6], a determination of these coefficients must be achieved with an accuracy between 0.5% and 1%. This is very difficult since quantum noise alone will result in a quantity of more than 100 kR for each measured value. So it is necessary to have a high signal–noise ratio; all of which reinforces the impossibility of using radioisotopes as a source of radiation for tomographic scanning. Variations or fluctuations in the voltage applied to the emitter tube are also not admissible.

If we use an absolute scale of debilitation there will be a series of practical problems, so it is advisable to start from the fundamental equation that explains the extent of absorption of x-rays by any material, to obtain a scale of relative debilitation coefficients. This allows us to reference the measurements to a suitable material with a known coefficient, such as water, and thus express the values of different substances found by the x-ray beam in positive or negative values up to a limit. As stated before, actual devices use a scale from +1000 to −1000.

X-ray absorption is determined by the following expression:

$$I = I_0 e^{-\int \mu dx},$$

where:

I = photon intensity received by the detector after passing through the body;
I_0 = the intensity emitted by the x-ray tube in the linear direction;
μ = the attenuation or absorption coefficient; and
d = the thickness of the object.

This is mathematically valid [7] in the case of monochromatic radiation and in very thin layers, which does not prevent the consideration of the attenuating effect of a set of thin layers placed in line one behind the other in the direction of the radiation beam. The net result is a photon intensity determined by the sum of the coefficients of each of the layers, which does not permit one to calculate the attenuation coefficient of each of the layers *per se*. This is shown in figure 15.3, which shows a similar total attenuation in two sets of three distinct layers.

These results can be graphed and expressed mathematically as shown in figure 15.4, in which the intensity collected after passing through the five layers can be seen. This is determined by the debilitation producing all of them, and is expressed as follows:

$$I = I_0 e^{-\int (\mu a da + \mu b db + \mu c dc + \mu d dd + \mu e de)}.$$

Thus, with conventional radiology information is only obtainable on the morphology of the tissue, and not on the attenuation ability of each layer or stratum, since the photonic intensity received informs us of the total attenuation and not the partial components. Now, if that same narrow collimated beam is used to traverse only a single layer, we will have information relating to the absorbent properties of the material that makes up the stratum. If we then make a displacement of the x-ray beam toward a contiguous zone of different composition (the shaded area in figure 15.5), we will see that the new information will, in addition,

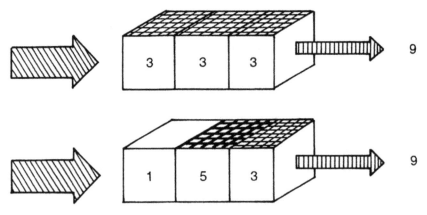

Figure 15.3. Identical total attenuation effect in materials with different densities.

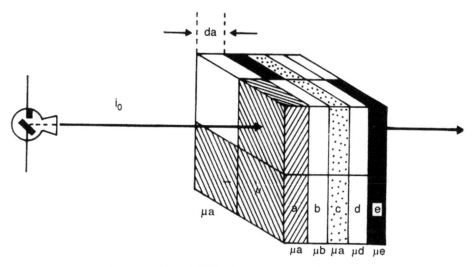

Figure 15.4. Total debilitation after crossing five layers.

correspond to the variation of the absorption properties. This is shown in figure 15.5, in which we can see that by knowing the emitted intensity, the value of received intensity (collected in the detector) and the thickness of the layer, we can calculate the corresponding coefficient (μb) from the above equation, in which the coefficient μd has been replaced by the value μb.

15.4 The axial irradiation procedure

If the block shown in figure 15.5 is subjected to irradiation with x-rays, in the axial rather than perpendicular manner, the beam only applies to a single stratum for that time. If in addition a displacement occurs corresponding to that of the CT x-ray tube, we may have a situation like the one shown in figure 15.6.

For simplicity we only shown the presence of four beams of radiation which can be considered as a system of equations, consisting of four equations with four

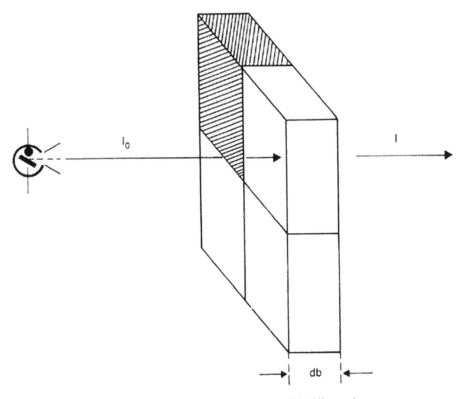

Figure 15.5. A collimated beam on a layer with different tissues.

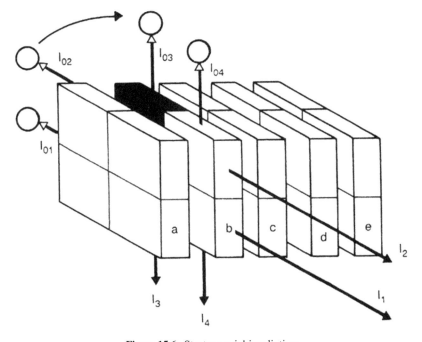

Figure 15.6. Stratum axial irradiation.

unknowns of photon intensity, which are the coefficients of debilitation of the four equal parts into which the layer is divided ($I_{01} + \cdots I_{04}$) (see figure 15.7).

The photon intensity equation becomes:

$$I = I_{01}e^{-(\mu_{11}+\mu_{21})}.$$

Then

$$\mu_1 + \mu_2 = \ln \frac{I}{I_0}.$$

So the system of equations is

$$\begin{array}{c}\mu_1 + \mu_2 = A \\ \mu_3 + \mu_4 = B \\ \mu_1 + \mu_3 = C \\ \mu_3 + \mu_4 = D\end{array}$$

which allows us to theoretically calculate the four coefficients required. Then the computer system can reconstruct an image on the screen, assigning shades of gray or colors to the numerical values calculated.

15.5 The procedure for calculated attenuation coefficents

The mathematical procedure to find the values of absorption of radiation can be performed in three ways.

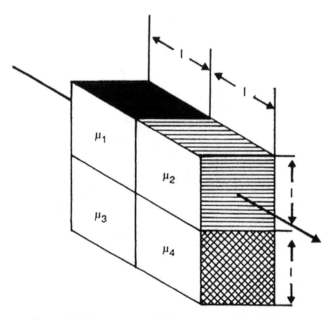

Figure 15.7. Four strata of different absorption coefficients.

15.5.1 Algebraic procedure

The algebraic procedure consists in solving the equations of the system once complete measurements have been taken and the values of *A*, *B*, *C* and *D* of the above equations have been obtained. These values correspond to the attenuation profiles of each projection. Figure 15.8 shows the assumed values of the coefficients of an equation system corresponding to the sum of the horizontal, vertical and diagonal attenuations.

15.5.2 The iterative or adaptive procedure

The algebraic system has the following drawback: a large number of equations need to be solved, because over 150 × 150 voxels are taken for a piece of biological tissue. Therefore, one should use a method that simplifies and shortens the measurement process. This method is called iterative, and its concepts are illustrated in figures 15.9 and 15.10.

The iterative procedure involves initially assuming values that satisfy some of the totals obtained. Thus, if a horizontal total is 8, 4 + 4 or 6 + 2 can validate this total. The next step is to verify which of these distributions satisfies not only the horizontal

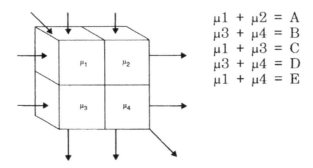

Figure 15.8. Five axial projections and their respective equations.

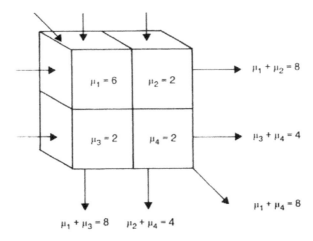

Figure 15.9. Values of absorption coefficient assumptions.

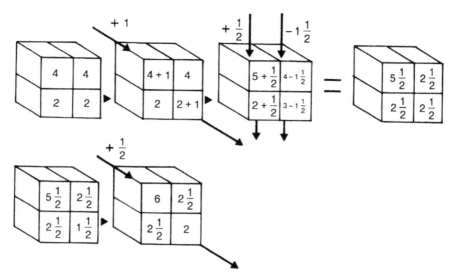

Figure 15.10. Development of the iterative process.

projections but also the diagonal and vertical. If the partial results are unsatisfactory, intermediate values of addition or subtraction will be assigned in each projection to ensure that the values satisfy all equations in the best possible way. This is the concept of iteration, although it appears to be longer, it is a more efficient way work with a computer.

To better understand the process let us assign supposed values to each coefficient: thus μ_1 and μ_2 have a value of 4, and μ_3 and μ_4 have a value of 2. These values satisfied the sum of the horizontal $\mu_1 + \mu_2 = 8$ and $\mu_3 + \mu_4 = 4$, but do not satisfy the diagonal sum of $\mu_1 + \mu_4 = 8$, therefore 1 is added to each diagonal value and these are compared with the measured values. The remaining contradiction indicates that it is necessary to introduce a new correction coefficient to ensure the appropriate vertical sums. Therefore 1/2 is added to the two vertical coefficients on the left, and the same value plus 1 is subtracted from the two vertical coefficients, i.e. subtract 1 and 1/2. The result obtained is not yet satisfactory so the value of 1/2 is added to the diagonal coefficients, which still show a lack in the resulting diagonal, which leads to the addition of another 1/2 to these diagonals. Finally note the excess in the horizontal and vertical amounts, as well as the diagonal not considered, i.e. ($\mu_2 + \mu_3$), so the last operation is to subtract 1/2 from μ_2 and μ_3, obtaining in this way the definitive values that satisfy all the equations. In practice the iterative process is carried out to have tolerable accuracy values. The fundamental defect of the iterative method is that it requires the total number of measurements to begin the adaptation; this is why the image would only be available after a certain time.

15.5.3 Back-projection

The method which is used providing the best practical results was introduced to the application of medical images by Kuhl, and essentially consists of returning to the

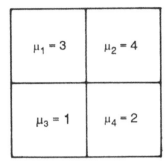

Figure 15.11. Actual values of absorption coefficients.

matrix of each retrieved profile [8], adding the resulting values to the first estimated which correspond to a total in each projection. So, finally, the values obtained for each coefficient are subtracted from the sum of all real coefficients and this is divided by the number of elements minus one. A numerical example will clarify this concept.

If we have a block with four coefficients, as shown in figure 15.11, we start from the knowledge of the actual values, and thus logically we know the sum of each projection:

$$\mu_1 + \mu_2 = 7$$
$$\mu_3 + \mu_4 = 3.$$

With the resulting values of the horizontal projection, we form a new matrix in which we back-project the totals obtained, then we have:

$\mu'_1 = 7$	$\mu'_2 = 7$
$\mu'_3 = 3$	$\mu'_4 = 3$

Now with the vertical projection in each case, we obtain other values in addition to the above matrix

$$\mu_1 + \mu_3 = 4$$
$$\mu_2 + \mu_4 = 6.$$

When added to what has already been obtained in the chart we obtain:

$\mu'_1 = 7+4$	$\mu'_2 = 7+6$
$\mu'_3 = 3+4$	$\mu'_4 = 3+6$

Then the diagonal values are obtained in the direction of the original matrix, i.e.:

$$\mu_1 + l = 3$$
$$\mu_3 + \mu_2 = 5.$$
$$l + \mu_3 = 2$$

The following shows the direction of the diagonal projections:

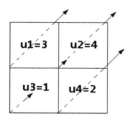

The values obtained are added to the values accumulated diagonally in the horizontal and vertical projections, yielding:

11+3	13+5
7+5	9+2

Then the diagonal sums are obtained in the other direction:

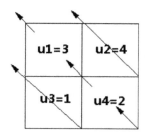

15-11

$$\mu_1 + \mu_4 = 5$$
$$\mu_2 + / = 4.$$
$$/ + \mu_3 = 1$$

Their values also added back diagonally to the last matrix obtained

$14 + 5$	$18 + 4$
$12 + 1$	$11 + 5$

The result of all the amounts determined by the various projections is subtracted from the value resulting from the sum of the real coefficients of the matrix with which we began the analysis:

$$\mu_1 + \mu_2 + \mu_3 + \mu_4 = 10.$$

So now the matrix has the following values

19-10	22-10
13-10	16-10

Dividing the result by 3 gives us the final result of the operation:

9/3	12/3
3/3	6/3

whereupon the correct results we already knew are obtained:

3	4
1	2

The process described is useful for understanding the mathematical meaning of the back-projection operation. However, it is clearer when a graphical explanation is examined, by obtaining simple profiles of attenuation and back-projecting on a graph that represent the field of view of the x-rays [9] in an equivalent of the axial section.

Graphic interpretation of back-projection
The purpose of axial scanning is to obtain a profile that can represent an object placed in the FOV, so that from any projection it has a similar profile. That is the case of a 'phantom' containing a sphere of material with higher density than the rest of the object, allowing the attenuation capacity of such a sphere to produce, from any angle, a profile with a notch corresponding to the sphere attenuation (see figure 15.12). In the case of introducing a sphere with smaller capacity x-ray absorption, we will have a different profile. Thus, the shape of the resulting profile is altered by an overshoot and no notch, compared to the previous case (see figure 15.13).

If the x-ray tube is shifted in an axial pattern, in the case of the phantom with a sphere of greater density in the center, we obtain a profile with a notch because the object of higher density absorbs radiation in greater quantities than the rest of the phantom, which produces an attenuation evidenced by the notch. The result is a set of similar profiles from any projection, as shown in figure 15.14.

Back-projection is to create an image using the profiles previously obtained [10], so that the grayscale values correspond to the densities that were found in the path of

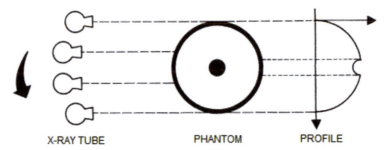

Figure 15.12. A phantom with an area of higher density.

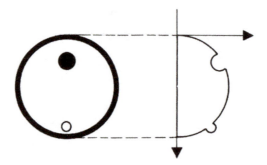

Figure 15.13. Profile resulting from the presence of different materials.

Technical Fundamentals of Radiology and CT

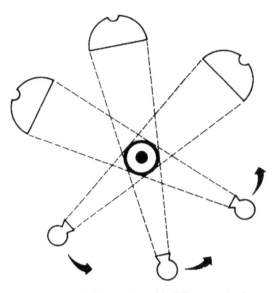

Figure 15.14. Similar profiles with different projections.

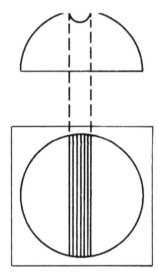

Figure 15.15. Back-projection of a single profile.

the radiation beam. Figure 15.15 shows a clear stripe corresponding to the greater attenuation; a region of grey corresponding to the uniform structure of the phantom and a black stripe for the object introduced in the phantom, which presents less attenuation. Thus the higher level of radiation received by the detector corresponds to more blackening. This image is the result of the back-projection of a single profile, obtained with the phantom between the tube and the detector. Figure 15.16 shows a result achieved with the combination of back-projection from different angles [11]. Strips obtained in the resulting image of different back-projections show that there is a point of union of the same shades of gray, which coincides with the geographic location of the corresponding sphere. So it is claimed that using the back-projection we can determine in which part of the FOV each object is located, even though the stripes extend along the entire length.

As the purpose of the CT is to obtain a representation of various structures [12], in an exact way and without artifacts, it is not acceptable to have stripes that represent the same density in different places of the image, where it is actually not the object that corresponds to the density. For this reason it is imperative to obtain a filtered image, i.e. delete all unnecessary information.

The need for filtration is clearly evident in figure 15.17 in which the result of a back-projection can be seen from all angles, in a variety of tomograms. With a simple phantom, which has one object of different density on one side, we obtain an image that places the object in the right place but appears in the image as a star and not a circle, as it should result in the final image, as shown in figure 15.18. A

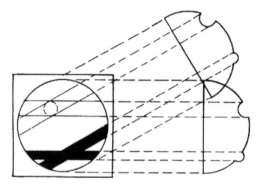

Figure 15.16. Location of objects using back-projection.

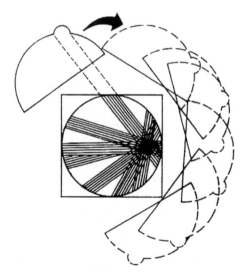

Figure 15.17. A circular object visible in a star shape.

Technical Fundamentals of Radiology and CT

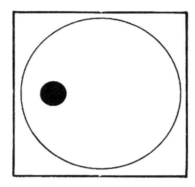

Figure 15.18. How the object should be displayed.

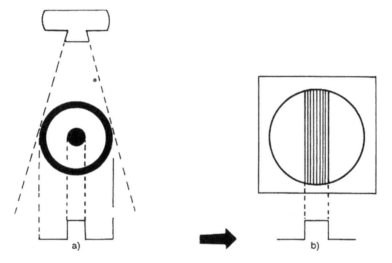

Figure 15.19. (a) A dense object in the center and (b) the obtained and back-projected profile.

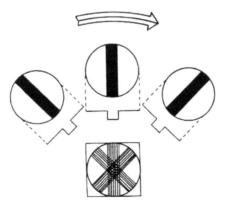

Figure 15.20. Axial profiles.

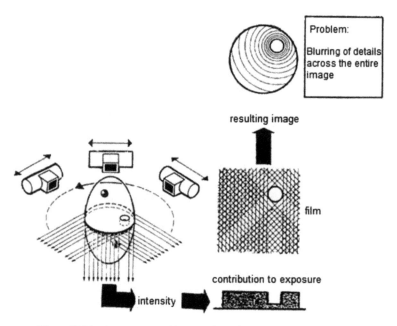

Figure 15.21. An uncorrected image of overlays. Courtesy of Siemens.

procedure of eliminating of the stripes and the stellate edges of the object should therefore be applied. The back-projection process is summarized in the following and filtration should be applied to the resulting image.

To obtain the axial projections of the object, the back-projection takes the same profile from different angles. Then, after the back-projection the result is an image that requires filtering, since it appears stellate as shown in figure 15.17, accompanied by fringes of lesser intensity, for all the objects, which represent the location of the denser object in the center of the circle, as shown in figure 15.19. Filtration is a corrective function that modifies the obtained profiles, so the back-projection produces an accentuation of the values of interest and the cancellation of the values that must be removed. The filtration is carried out by a convolution function [13].

Graphic interpretation of the convolution
To understand the process of obtaining the image through convolution or low frequency filtering of signals, the steps are described as follows. Print a film (or in the case of CT equipment, activate the system's optical display) [14] by means of a disperser that can convert intensity profiles into an equivalent brightness in stripes, as shown in figures 15.20 and 15.21; then moving the incident angle and the film to obtain a new dispersed image. Thus numerous overlapping images that form the layer are obtained.

Each profile contributes to the formation of the overall image, acting on the film from its angular location (see figure 15.20). The set of profiles will give an image where the sum of all shadow projections come together to reconstruct the object that is opaque to x-rays (the cylinder in the drawing), as shown in figure 15.21. This result is unsatisfactory due to the significant blurring of details, in particular for the entire outline of the object. To solve this problem we use convolution, which is the implementation of a corrective function [15] that will remove the blurred effect in the projections. For this we must give a prior step to the convolution; it consists of getting the logarithm of the values obtained. Applied to these results, the corrective function of convolution [16] manages to correct the assumed shadows of all structures of the object, before joining the total scattered image. This means modifying the profile so that the new image is favorably altered by the assumed shadows (favorable from the point of view of information and the shape of the image). As seen in figure 15.22, the corrective function alters the original profile in such a way that adding all the back-projections means the blurring will be removed [17].

Back-projections of filtered images
If you back-project the attenuation profiles obtained, after convoluting them graphically, the resulting images are very different to those obtained using simple back-projection of unconvolved profiles. A profile fixed by convolution presents positive and also negative displacement compared to the signal zero axis. Thus, the adopting of such profiles is equivalent to finding the objects with greater or lesser densities than the reference value (water). So joining all back-projected profiles from different directions in a single image produces an image with the blurring and the stripes along the entire object removed, and only thus is an exact reproduction of the

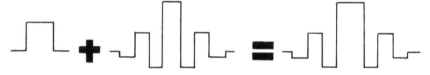

Figure 15.22. Applying the filtering function.

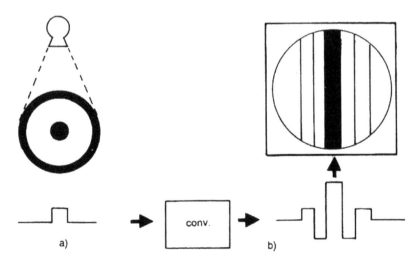

Figure 15.23. (a) Original profile and (b) convoluted and back-projected profile.

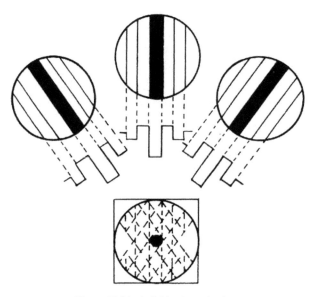

Figure 15.24. Axial back-projection.

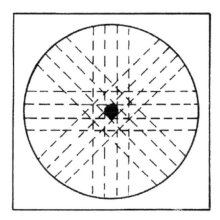

Figure 15.25. The image obtained by convoluted back-projection.

scanned object obtained [18]. Figure 15.23 shows the retrieved profile and its further convolution, giving rise to a clear image.

Now consider axial scans, with their respective profiles subsequently back-projected (see figure 15.24), then convolved and joined in a single, final image. The resulting image, as shown in figure 15.25, is free from artifacts and shaped edges like stars, and is much closer to the original shape [19] of the scanned object.

References

[1] Hounsfield G 1973 Computerized transverse axial scanning tomography. Part 1: description of system *Br. J. Radiol.* **46** 1016

[2] Pfeiler M and Schwierz G 1976 Conceptos modelo sobre la reproducción de las imágenes en la tomografía axial con computador *Electromédica* **1** 19–25

[3] Scudder H J 1978 Introduction to computer aided tomography *Proc. IEEE* **66** 628

[4] Hill K R 1976 EMI total body scanner: technical aspects *Br. J. Clin. Equip.* **1** 207–14

[5] Dummling K 1984 10 años de tomografía computarizada–visión retrospectiva *Electromédica* **1** 13–28

[6] Horn E 1978 X-ray computed tomography *Electron. Power* **24** 36–41

[7] Fineberg H 1979 Advances and dilemmas in computed tomography *Proc. IEEE* **67** 1272–3

[8] Randall R B 1977 *Application of B&K, Equipment to Frequency Analysis* (Nærum: Brüel and Kjaer)

[9] Herman G T 2009 *Fundamentals of Computerized Tomography: Image Reconstruction from Projections* (London: Springer)

[10] Peters T 2002 CT image reconstruction *AAPM Annual Meeting* (14–18 *July* 2002, *Montreal, Canada*) https://www.aapm.org/meetings/02AM/pdf/8372-23331.pdf

[11] Ewen K and Fisher P 1977 La exposición a la radiación útil y dispersa en la tomografía computarizada *Electromédica* **1** 8–16

[12] Kachelrieß M Basics of CT image reconstruction (*Erlangen, Germany*) www.dkfz.de/en/medphysrad/workinggroups/ct/ct_conference_contributions/BasicsOfCTImageReconstruction_Part1.pdf www.dkfz.de/en/medphysrad/workinggroups/ct/ct_conference_contributions/BasicsOfCTImageReconstruction_Part2.pdf

[13] Smith A W 1997 *The Scientist and Engineer's Guide to Digital Signal Processing* (San Diego, CA: California Technical Publishing) ch 25

[14] Kak A and Jakowats V 1975 Computerized tomography using video recorder fluoroscopic images *IEEE Trans. Biomed. Eng.* **24** 157

[15] General Electric Medical Systems 1986 CT traveler (module Il) *Sales Data*

[16] Compagnie Generale de Radiologie 1980 ND 8000 physical aspects *TDM Information*

[17] Webb W R, Brant W E and Major N M 2014 *Fundamentals of Body CT* (Philadelphia, PA: Saunders)

[18] GE Healthcare 2014 Rapid and precise TAVI planning with Revolution* CT *GE Healthcare* www3.gehealthcare.co.uk/en-gb/products/categories/computed_tomography/revolution_ct/clinical_case_-_rapid_and_precise_tavi_planning_with_revolution_ct

[19] Homma N 2011 *Theory and Applications of CT Imaging and Analysis* (Rijeka: InTech)

IOP Publishing

Technical Fundamentals of Radiology and CT

Guillermo Avendaño Cervantes

Chapter 16

Mathematical analysis of convolution

16.1 Introduction

The algorithm for the reconstruction of one section of a two-dimensional square, from a sequence of a one-dimensional profile of x-rays, is based on the theorem of two-dimensional analysis by Fourier. This theorem establishes that the Fourier transform of a one-dimensional projection of an object is identical to the corresponding central section of the two-dimensional Fourier transform of the object [1]. That is, the Fourier transform of x-rays from the step explorer profile at a given angle, is identical to the value of the Fourier transform of the two-dimensional section of the explored plane along the line passing through the center of the transform at the same angle. However, before handling the specific concepts of the convolution applied to CT, it is necessary to give an introduction to the Fourier transform and the convolution of functions.

Fourier analysis allows the determination of the component frequencies of sinusoidal forms [2], coupled with giving a specific signal as the result. In other words, any signal or function such as that can be obtained through radiation profiles, after the process of photonics sensing of the collimated beam, can be divided into numerous sinusoidal components of a certain amplitude A, initial phase Φ and a certain frequency f.

However, it is necessary to represent each sinusoidal component in a way that ensures its appropriate mathematical management. This is usually represented by a wave which merges with a single x-axis angular value and time (see figure 16.1). Therefore, in Fourier analysis, the representation of each component is shown as the vector sum of two counter-rotating vectors, as shown in figure 16.1 where the vector is presented at time zero.

It can be seen that as the wave travels along the time axis, the counter-rotating vectors always give a value on the real axis on the right side of the figure, as if the

doi:10.1088/978-0-7503-1212-7ch16

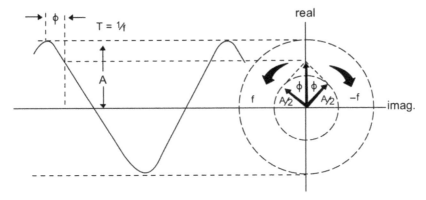

Figure 16.1. Sinusoidal and vector representations.

wave is perpendicular to the paper. Both forms contained in the mathematical figure are related by:

$$A = \cos\theta = \frac{A}{2}(e^{j\phi} + e^{-j\phi}),$$

where
$\theta = 2\pi ft + \Phi$,
A = amplitude;
f = frequency of the component;
φ = phase angle with respect to zero; and
θ = linear variation with time of the phase angle.

All this can be better understood if we move the graphic/mathematical representation of the vectors into a complex plane, as shown in figure 16.2. The equal vectors are displaced on both sides of the imaginary values and have a modular F value. Then its components are:

$$a = F \cos\theta$$
$$b = F \sin\theta,$$

with

$$F = \sqrt{(a^2 + b^2)}$$

and the angle

$$\theta = \arctan^{-1}\left(\frac{b}{a}\right).$$

Since the vectors have a mathematical representation of

$$F = a \pm jb$$

Technical Fundamentals of Radiology and CT

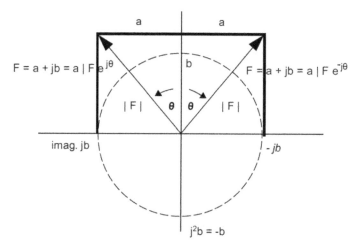

Figure 16.2. Vector components.

we obtain

$$F = |F|(\cos\theta + j\sin\theta),$$

and using the relationship of Euler

$$\cos\theta + j\sin\theta = e^{j\theta}$$

$$F = |F|e^{j\theta}.$$

As the product of two vectors is known to be equal to the product of their amplitudes and the resulting angle is the sum of their angles, it follows that multiplication by a unit vector does not affect the amplitude, but adds to the angle phase value equal to 0, that is, it rotates the vector in angle φ.

16.2 Fourier analysis

Now we proceed to obtain expressions that allow us to calculate any component of a signal studied at the same time, the total value corresponding to the sum of all components. This is achieved on the basis of considering each sinusoidal component as a vector [3].

So we have a periodic function

$$g(t) = g(t + nt),$$

where

t = time; and
n = any integer including 1 and negative values.

This periodic function can be represented by a sum of s rotating vectors, Kf_1 equally spaced frequencies, where $f_1 = 1/T$ and K is an integer, thus the kth component can be obtained from

$$G(f_k) = \frac{1}{T}\int_{-T/2}^{T/2} g(t)e^{-2\pi jkt}dt,$$

where $fk = kf_1$. Through the latter equation can be obtained or extracted $g(t)$ and the contained components which each rotate at a frequency fk. The real position of each vector at any time t can be obtained by multiplying the initial value $g(fk)$, by the opposite rotary vector

$$g(t) = \sum_{k=-\infty}^{k=\infty} G(f_k) e^{-2\pi fkt}.$$

So the overall signal $g(t)$ is the vector sum of all vectors in their current position.

The sum of complex values $G(fk)$, is known as the spectrum components of $g(t)$, and there is an amplitude and phase (or real and imaginary equivalent) associated with each; therefore, a complete representation requires three dimensions, as shown in figure 16.3.

In the most general case, when the space $1/T$ between the harmonics tends to zero, then the penultimate equation tends to take the overall value

$$G(f) = \int_{-\infty}^{\infty} g(t) e^{-j2\pi fkt} dt$$

and the last equation tends to

$$G(t) = \int_{-\infty}^{\infty} g(f) e^{-j2\pi fkt} df.$$

Both equations are called a Fourier transform pair. The first is called the direct Fourier transform. Both are almost symmetrical, differing only in the sign of e.

When the function is sampled in both time and frequency, with both the time signal and the frequency spectrum made periodic, the transformed pair is known as a pair of discrete Fourier transforms, meaning:

$$G(t) = \frac{1}{N} \sum_{n=0}^{n=1} g(n) e^{-\frac{j2\pi Kn}{K}},$$

the value corresponding to the forward transform.

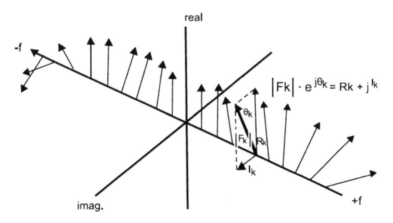

Figure 16.3. Spectrum components $g(t)$.

Meanwhile the inverse transform takes the form:

$$g(n) = \frac{1}{N}\sum_{n=0}^{n=1} G(k)e^{-\frac{j2\pi Kn}{K}},$$

where K refers to the frequency fK, and n to the time; meanwhile tn is the number of samples N in time, i.e. the given number of frequencies. The pair of discrete transforms has the advantage of replacing a finite sum of an infinite length, which facilitates its use in digital computing.

In 1965 a method was published that significantly reduces the number of arithmetic operations, and has revolutionized the field of signal analysis. This method, known as the fast Fourier transform [4] is a very practical and useful algorithm used in computing and CT.

16.3 Convolution

One of the most important properties of the Fourier transform is the fact that it can achieve a transform of the convolution in a multiplication. We need to define the convolution of two functions to understand the process of implementation in CT. The convolution of functions, one with time $f(t)$ and the other with $g(t)$, is mathematically defined as:

$$g(t) = \int_{-\infty}^{\infty} f(\tau)h(t-\tau)d\tau,$$

which is represented as follows:

$$g(t) = f(t)*h(t),$$

where the asterisk (*) means convolved with.

One of the major applications of this relationship is in the case where $f(t)$ represents the input signal of a physical system, and $h(t)$ represents the impulse response of the system. Therefore, $g(t)$ will be the system output [5]. The physical meaning can be seen in figure 16.4.

In figure 16.5 (a) represents a time signal $f(t)$ and (b) applies to the impulse response of the actual physical system. It is assumed that each point in $f(t)$ can be considered with an impulse (delta function) weighted by $f(t)$ at that point; each of these pulses excites a response pulse.

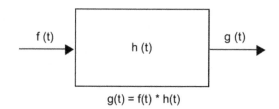

Figure 16.4. The convolution response of a physical system.

Technical Fundamentals of Radiology and CT

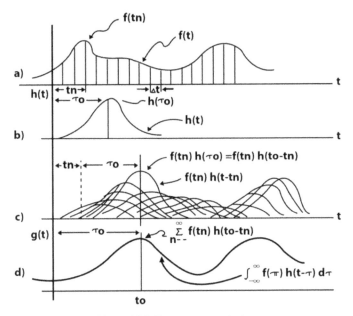

Figure 16.5. Response convolution.

The output signal at time t, $g(t)$, is the sum of all these response pulses, each delayed by an appropriate interval from the excitation time until measurement. Because each point of the response curve is a sum of components which are being excited at different times, it is necessary to integrate over a fictitious variable time.

It can be seen that the peak value in (c) occurs in $t_0 = t_n + \tau_0$, in which τ_0 is shown in (b) as the value at the peak time of the pulse response in the physical system. The peak value is evident, i.e.

$$f(t_n)h(t_0 - t_n)$$

and thus at any time t the value of the response is equal to

$$f(t_n)h(t - t_n).$$

The response time τ_0 from the signal applied at time τ_n can be $g_n(\tau_0)$ and so the total response at time τ_0 is equal to the sum of all responses excited at various times:

$$g(t_0) = \sum_{n=-\infty}^{n=\infty} gn(t_0) = \sum_{n=-\infty}^{n=\infty} f(t_n)h(t_0 - t_n).$$

At time t the answer is

$$g(t) = \sum_{n=-\infty}^{n=\infty} f(tn)h(t - t_n).$$

This function in the limit when $d\tau$ tends to zero, approaches the equation:

$$g(t) = f(t)*h(t).$$

All previous explanations refer to two real functions, but this can convolve complex functions, for example two spectral frequencies

$$F(f)*H(f) = \int_{\infty}^{\infty} F(\theta)H(f - \theta)d\theta,$$

but since the $F(f)$ and $H(f)$ are complex variables, the multiplication is now of complex type (the multiplication sum of amplitudes and phases).

16.3.1 The convolution theorem

The convolution theorem states that in the Fourier transform (forward and reverse), the convolution becomes a multiplication. If

$$G(t) = F\langle g(t)\rangle.$$

The direct Fourier transform of $g(t)$ is

$$F(t) = F\langle f(t)\rangle$$

$$H(t) = F\langle h(t)\rangle$$

and if

$$G(t) = f(t)*h(t)$$

then

$$G(f) = F(t)H(f).$$

This means that the Fourier transform of a function of time, which is the result of the convolution of two functions, is the product of the Fourier transforms of the two functions.

16.4 Application to CT

The previously developed mathematical tools allow us to understand what was initially raised: a convolution in space is equivalent to a multiplication in Fourier space [6], therefore, to handle functions in Fourier space, they can be expressed in terms of their spatial frequencies rather than in terms of their spatial coordinates [7]. This means that through convolution, one can improve an image (the attenuation profile function), by applying a correction function (the equivalent to a filtering frequency). So the frequency analysis is adequate to describe the convolution used in CT.

The latter can be better understood if we analyze the reconstruction of an image from attenuation profiles corresponding to numerous individual projections in graphical form. It follows that to reconstruct an image by means of projections, in addition to the desired image of the layer, smearing also appears. This can be removed by filtration of low frequencies, which is achieved mathematically by convolution.

The concept of graphical filtering of low frequencies is illustrated in figure 16.6, in which the filtering effect on low frequencies of semi-closed eyes of the observer is shown.

Technical Fundamentals of Radiology and CT

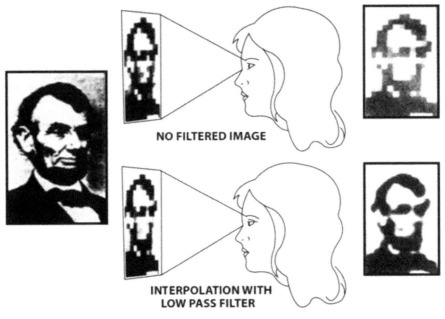

Figure 16.6. The filter effect of semi-closed eyes. Courtesy of Siemens.

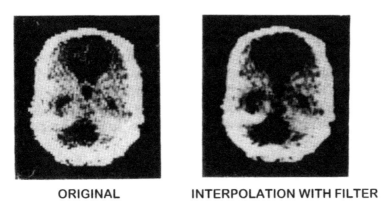

Figure 16.7. Filtering of a brain image. Courtesy of Siemens.

The head of President Lincoln, converted into an image based on pixels, is observed in the upper part of the figure with eyes open, the result can be seen on the right. The same image seen with eyes semi-closed (filtration), allows a different result, in which a better image is obtained, because in the final result the effect of pixels is not as noticeable. Comparing the two panels of figure 16.7, the result of low frequency filtration is evident [8]. A computerized tomogram of a skull, made with a computer, in which the pixels are seen in the resulting figure, is greatly improved by image processing based on low-pass filtering.

References

[1] Compagnie Generale de Radiologie 1977 Basic principles in tomodensitometry

[2] Avendaño G 1979 Algunos aspectos matemático-ingenieriles de la tomografía axial computarizada *Electromedicina* **1** 2–19

[3] Randall R B 1977 *Application of B&K Equipment to Frequency Analysis* (Nærum: Brüel and Kjaer)

[4] Sheep L and Logan B 1986 The Fourier reconstruction of a head section *IEEE Trans. Nucl. Sci.* **21** 21

[5] Kak A 1979 Computerized tomography with x-ray emission and ultrasound sources *Proc. IEEE* **67** 1245

[6] General Electric Medical Systems 1987 CT traveler (module III) *Sales Data*

[7] Tretiak O 1979 Noise limitation in x-ray computed tomography *J. Comput. Assist. Tomogr.* **2** 477

[8] Dreike P and Boyd D 1976 Convolution reconstruction of fan beam projections *Comput. Graph. Image Process* **5** 459

IOP Publishing

Technical Fundamentals of Radiology and CT

Guillermo Avendaño Cervantes

Chapter 17

Forms of exploration

17.1 Introduction

The principle of imaging in CT is based on a collimated beam of radiation that is applied to the object, and a diametrically opposite detector that picks up the radiation weakened by the attenuation of the scanned object. This system is composed of an x-ray tube and a detector that move around the object in solidarity, first in a linear motion and then turning gradually to go completely around the object.

Currently this only serves to explain the principle of exploration, since there are no actual devices that work based on this principle. The original model has been improved and there are now four basic modes of exploration, referred to as four generations. Some authors disagree with the classification into generations, since according to their way of understanding the technology, a generation is not necessarily better that the previous one, since manufacturers use different generations. It is perhaps preferable to speak of scanning modes and principles [1].

17.2 Principle 1 (translation–rotation)

Principle 1 corresponds to the basic CT scan mode description. The collimated beam starts at one point and moves linearly along the entire structure, as shown in figure 17.1. At the end of the second translation another twist or rotation occurs, which gives the other name used to define this principle, translation–rotation. After completing 180 translations and rotations, the scan ends. Thus different tissues contained in the stratum have been covered from all angles and all respective attenuation profiles have been obtained. Figures 17.2 and 17.3 summarize object scanning using a collimated beam, demonstrating the so-called first generation or principle 1.

This process takes between 4.5 min and 5 min, so it cannot be used for body scans [2], since respiratory movement, the movements of the heart and the peristalsis of some organs in the body would produce very disturbing effects or artifacts in

doi:10.1088/978-0-7503-1212-7ch17

Technical Fundamentals of Radiology and CT

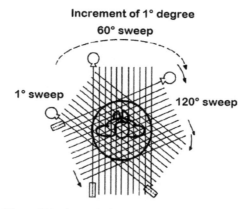

Figure 17.1. A translation–rotation collimated beam.

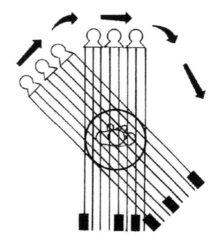

Figure 17.2. Principle 1 or first generation CT.

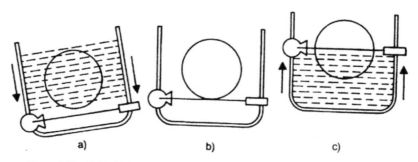

Figure 17.3. (a) End of translation. (b) Rotating degree. (c) Another translation.

the images. It became imperative to reduce the times of exploration to avoid such problems, also because the irradiation on the patient was of a high value over the long scan duration, and therefore dangerous for both patients and staff. This series of problems led equipment designers to think about how to use the radiation emitted more efficiently and devise a way to produce shorter scans. The result was what is now known as the second generation or principle 2: translation–rotation with multiple detectors.

17.3 Principle 2 (translation–rotation)

By taking advantage of x-ray emission in the form of divergent radiation from the tube to the detector, the collimation is reduced or eliminated [3], so that radiation can reach various detectors placed at the other end. The number of detectors is variable, in figure 17.4 we show three, but it may be possible to accommodate up to 60 with a good electronic and mechanical design.

The second generation uses a method similar to that used in the first. The linear translation of the irradiation system along with the set of detectors is carried out, and after completing the exploration of the object, a turn of one degree at a time occurs (figure 17.5). Completing the scan shows a remarkable reduction in time for the collection of the same attenuation profiles compared to principle 1. The principle 2 scanning system has a duration of approximately 2 min.

A further reduction of the time of exploration allowed by the second generation involves using a very high number of detectors, which are, of course, limited by the physical dimensions. Also, it is not possible to perform the movement more quickly,

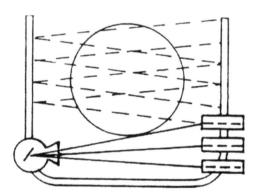

Figure 17.4. Translation–rotation with three detectors.

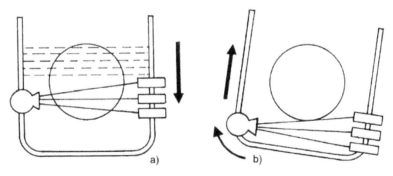

Figure 17.5. (a) Translation. (b) Turn and new exploration.

Technical Fundamentals of Radiology and CT

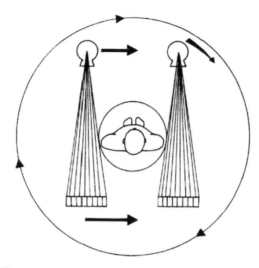

Figure 17.6. Translation–rotation with multiple detectors.

because a real device has the great limitation of the inertia of the movements of the whole system [4]. The fixed tube and detectors need to start from a stationary position with high inertia and speed up to a constant and harmonic speed to be able to collect the data without interference or noise. Then the system needs stop completely before performing a rotation or turn of the required grade and then restart the sequence of operations described, without loosening or producing vibrations. Attaining such mechanical properties is very complex and it is almost impossible to manufacture such a device. Figure 17.6 shows a representation of the different beams of radiation over a system of multiple detectors that comply with the second generation.

17.4 Principle 3 (rotation–rotation)

The technical problems that prevent the system from attaining the necessary speed to obtain images in shorter times, were famously solved with the rotation–rotation system or third generation/principle 3, in which the translational movement is abandoned to perform only a rotational movement of the tube together with the set of detectors (see figure 17.7). This movement is possible because the x-ray tube emits a fan beam of radiation projected at an angle of the order of 40–50°, not a collimated beam.

This fan beam falls, after traversing the object, on a set of detectors in an arc located in the bottom of a circular sector. Thus, in a single full turn, the radiation covers all points of the object from different projections, which achieves the goal of obtaining the desired profiles in a very short time, of the order of seconds. This allows the possibility of studying parts of the body that have slow movements. An important feature of this system is the fact that the tube can work in a modality for pulsed emission of radiation, activating and blocking radiation each 0.5° or 1° angle, so the wear of the tube is reduced and the patient is irradiated less.

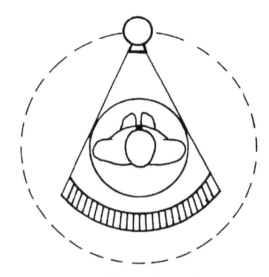

Figure 17.7. Rotation–rotation.

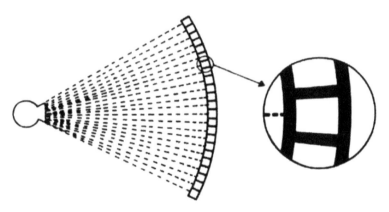

Figure 17.8. Collimated radiation detectors and spacing.

The fan does not consist of a bundle that occupies the entire volume of the arc, because it is only necessary to receive radiation in the detectors and not between them. The dead space between the detectors does not provide any information (see figure 17.8). Obviously depending on how many detectors there are the arc [5], more information will be obtained in less time with this system.

17.5 Principle 4 (rotation–rotation)

This technique is achieved through the exclusive movement of the tube rotating inside a ring of fixed detectors, the tube moves in a circle with a radius less than the radius of the arc (see figure 17.9). The radiation emitted by the tube is a fan beam and is picked up by the detectors placed along the ring around the patient [6]. This system allows one to obtain scan times similar to those of the third generation, and in comparison principle 4 has some advantages, but also some disadvantages [7].

Technical Fundamentals of Radiology and CT

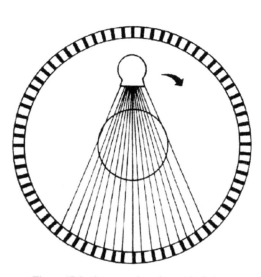

Figure 17.9. A system based on principle 4.

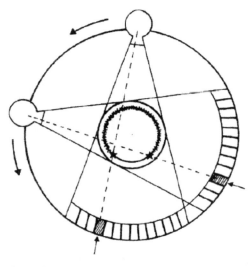

Figure 17.10. Circular artifacts produced by an unadjusted detector.

The most significant advantage is related to the fact that in the third generation, a mismatch or bad function from any detector (cell) will cause a response different from the other detectors, and this manifests as a circular artifact in the image. This is the result of having a beam out of adjustment in tangent to a circle that is formed with the movement of the tube–detector arrangement; the circle appears in the reconstructed image, as shown in figure 17.10.

Another advantage of the ring with fixed detectors system, is that when you only move the tube, scanning times are very short and above all the mechanics of the system are significantly simplified. However, the disadvantages of the system are also significant: a greater spacing between detectors decreasing the capture and subsequent use of attenuated rays. Also, this system required larger distances

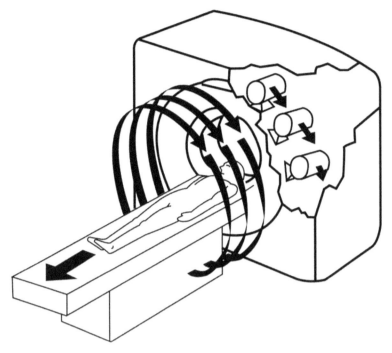

Figure 17.11. A helical rotation system.

between the patient and the detectors, so the spatial resolution and the dose are reduced [8].

17.6 Principle 5 (helical rotation)

Contemporary devices use an innovative initial scan system concept, with rotation of the tube in a gantry resulting in a helix-shaped path through the simultaneous action produced by longitudinal displacement of the table along with the rotation of the tube (see figure 17.11). Thus the patient is explored more quickly and the number of cuts obtained is higher. This system incorporates several rings with detectors, so is called a multicut system.

17.7 Multislice helical CT

Helical CT devices differ from conventional devices, to take advantage of the continuous rotation of the detectors and the x-ray tube, synchronized with the continuous movement of the table inside the gantry. Such a multislice helical scan system allows full body examination in one patient apnea (the time it takes the patient to holds his/her breath once), with some advantageous features:
- Achievement of very good diagnostic detail due to a resolution below 0.4 mm.
- A very low turnaround time of about 0.33 s.
- The the axial resolution (axis z) can be optimized, which grants the possibility of exploring volumes with submillimeter resolution, as already indicated.

- The device uses a system of detector multilines (up to 128) based on the latest generation of ultra-fast response solid-state transducers, allowing a wide choice of slice thicknesses.
- The detectors are built based on the solid-state principle with the most advanced technology and are designed to form a matrix, reducing the dose reaching the patient and allowing the faster scan times mentioned.
- Image quality is improved by increasing the signal–noise ratio.
- Excellent image quality, high efficiency of dose and the possibility of maximum coverage of the volume to explore can be achieved.
- Helical CT images have better spatial resolution as data is captured continuously and so the images can overlap. In conventional CT, pathological details may not be visible in the images because they are located just between two cuts, but with the reconstruction of transverse overlapping images the details will be visible in the center cut.
- The overlap is not necessarily the result of a higher dose of radiation, rather it is the result of the greater complexity in the mathematical processing of the reconstruction [9].
- Better images of anatomical structures are achieved, including those involved in respiratory movements, resulting in detailed critical studies of the thorax, abdomen and pelvis in general; and also excellent images of other body regions where there are no problems with movement such as the skull, spine and limbs.
- The intracranial arteries and smaller branches of coronary arteries can be observed, along with studies of pulmonary vessels, renal and mesenteric studies, and enteroclysis (a major study that takes place in the intestines, with administration of a contrast medium through a nasogastric tube), and determination of the state of tissues at the submillimeter level can be performed. These studies are not possible with other diagnostic imaging procedures.
- Very detailed studies as intravascular endoscopy, bronchoscopy and pielouretroscopy are possible.

To achieve these impressive results, important technological advances have been developed for modern helical multidetector devices, to achieve continuous high-speed movement without imperfections that could affect the quality of the images, and allowing the capture of electrical signals on a rotating basis without involving large numbers of cables, as in conventional CT. Along with the continuous reception of data as they are acquired, this forces these systems to have high-level algorithms and the best support software possible, and a high storage capacity to process in parallel what is being acquired in real time [10].

Some multislice helical CT devices introduce extra collimation of the additional detectors to offset the loss of spatial resolution. This causes a portion of the x-rays to not constitute a signal source, so the system requires an increase in the filament current tube (mA) to achieve the same signal intensity. This generates the disadvantage of increasing the radiation dose to the patient. These devices are classified as multislice helical CT with high resolution. The main advantage of this technology is that it can analyze a large amount of tissue. With modern devices the entire body can be explored in one apnea.

There are two basic concepts to be specified for multislice CT scanning, namely:
1. The beam displacement factor.
2. The displacement of cutting factor (pitch).

The first factor relates the movement of the patient table—for each 360° revolution—with the width of the x-ray beam. For example, for a matrix element of 16 detectors with a 1.25 mm width each, when all the detectors are used, the beam width will be 1.25 mm $\times$ 16 = 20 mm, if the table movement is 20 mm, factor beam displacement is 20 mm/20 mm = 1.0. If the same device uses only 8 detectors, the beam width will be 10 mm (8 $\times$ 1.25 mm = 10 mm) and the beam displacement factor is 20 mm/10 mm = 2.0.

The displacement of the cutting factor (or pitch) in helical CT is the movement of the patient bed for each 360° helical turn, divided by the slice thickness. The pitch determines the separation of the coils, so a 10 mm s^{-1} table movement, if each spin lasts 1 s and the thickness cut is 10 mm, corresponds to a pitch of 1 or, when expressed as a proportion, a pitch rate of 1:1. If the slice thickness was 5 mm, with the same displacement speed we obtain a value of pitch = (10 mm)/5 mm = 2, then the pitch rate is 2:1. So pitch = 1 means that there is a table translation equivalent to the slice thickness (produced by collimation) per rotation of the tube in the gantry. Pitch = 2 states that there is a shift of a double slice thickness per rotation of the tube on the gantry. The higher the value of the pitch, the more the helix is stretched, the coverage of exploration is greater, and there is less radiation to the patient, but with the disadvantage of lower quality images. In practice the beam displacement factor is typically 1.0. Multislice CT is available with 4, 8 or 16 simultaneous cuts at the same time, whereas conventional technology allows only one.

To assess the effectiveness of the system in relation to the acquisition of multislice images, the rate of cuts per rotation of 360° is defined, this is known as the slice acquisition rate (SAR). For the SAR it is necessary to consider the time of rotation. If the turnaround time is, for example, 1 s/360°, the SAR is equal to the number of cuts for every 360° explored.

The studied tissue volume is represented by the coverage in the shaft direction of movement, that is, along the z-axis. A mathematical expression that determines the coverage scanned volume is then set

$$Z = \text{SAR} \times W \times T \times B,$$

where
$Z = z$-axis coverage;
SAR = number of cuts/rotation time in seconds;
W = width of cut in mm;
T = time of analysis; and
B = beam displacement factor.

References

[1] Kreel L and Meire H 1977 The diagnostic process: a comparison of scanning techniques *Br. Med. J* **2** 809

[2] General Electric Medical Systems 1987 CT traveler *Sales Data*

[3] TDM 1979 ND 8OOO un tomodensitometre neuro radiologique (Compagnie General de Radiologie)

[4] General Electric Medical Systems 1986 CT/T technology continuum: technical performance of the CT/T system *Technical Booklet*

[5] Scharl P, Peter F and Weckesser W D 1979 Problems in the display of CT images by the use of television and photography *Electromédica* **2** 62–71

[6] General Electric Medical Systems 1897 GE fast-scan CT: a whole new generation *Sales Data* ch 2

[7] Ulla M and García R 2008 Tomografía computada multislice de 64 pistas: ¿Cómo, cuándo y por qué? *Rev. Hosp. Ital. B. Aires* **28** 28

[8] CENETEC 2009 Tomografía computarizada *Guía Tec* No. 6

[9] Csendes G P, Sanhueza S A and Aldana V H 2006 Aplicaciones de la tomografía computada multidetector en el estudio del intestino delgado *Rev. Hosp. Clín. Univ. Chile* **17** 279

[10] DEGIEM 2012 Rx-15 Tomógrafo computarizado de 64 cortes *Especificaciones Técnicas Código*

IOP Publishing

Technical Fundamentals of Radiology and CT

Guillermo Avendaño Cervantes

Chapter 18

Equipment for CT

18.1 Introduction

A complete system for CT must have a set of components that allows the desired images to be obtained in the most efficient way possible. We must define what is wanted or required in a CT system. Schematically it is intended that a system can perform the following tests:
- Scans to reconstruct images of the head or body.
- Obtaining anatomical images in a variety of positions and planes: positions such as decubitus, prone and supine; and planes such as axial, coronal and sagittal (although scanning is performed only axially).
- Obtaining images of any type of patient (from children to adults 50 cm in diameter and 210 kg in weight).

Although the devices were initially designed for limited purposes, such as those manufactured for cervical or cranial studies and specific research, subsequently developed systems are used for multiple studies such as those mentioned above.

Whatever the application of the CT device, it must comply with some basic technical requirements:
- Obtaining optimal image quality.
- A short time for image reconstruction allowing a high rate of introduction of patients.
- Maximum capacity management and playback.
- Technical reliability and maintenance.

The technological research and improvements introduced in contemporary computers have been directed toward the aforementioned purposes, in compliance with the stated requirements, benefitting both patients and the owners of the devices.

Any system must have:
- An examination table and gantry.
- A radiation generator system and its control.

doi:10.1088/978-0-7503-1212-7ch18 18-1 © IOP Publishing Ltd 2016

- A detection system and computer processing.
- System image display and diagnostics.
- Components for records, files and documentation.

Basic elements that can be extended to obtain greater advantages are valuable. We can increase the capacity of the basic memory, include additional consoles and, in particular, take advantage of the growing possibilities of software for many diagnostic applications.

18.2 The table

The scan table must have some important features [1] (see figure 18.1). The table movements, both horizontal displacement and lifting, must be highly accurate, allowing repeated measurements with the same or other patients in the same anatomical regions. Therefore, the table must have control software for movement, with very precise requirements for its parameters. Motor movements must be computerized with hydraulic control for lifting and the patient must be positioned exactly within the gantry, and there must simultaneously be the ability to suddenly discontinue the process due to emergencies.

In most modern systems, the table performs its movement synchronized with patient displacement and tube rotation. This determines a helical trajectory, where the pitch concept is applied. The table should also generally allow easy access and removal of patients.

18.3 Requirements for the table

The levels required for the movement of the table should be the following:
- Vertical displacement between 45 cm and 100 cm relative to the floor.
- Motorized displacement horizontally of at least 1000 mm with an accuracy of +0 to −1 mm per 2 mm increments.
- At least two-speed horizontal scrolling.

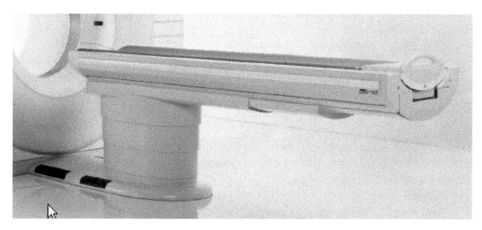

Figure 18.1. The table of a CT system. Courtesy of Siemens.

Controls governed by the software need to control the table so that the table movements are combined with the gantry, thus activation movements or changes in the inclination of the gantry are avoided. Each kind of table must have a control panel, located on either side of it, for selecting the values of height, lateral displacement increases and gantry tilt positioning lights (which can be a laser beam).

A helical scan acquires information continuously as the patient is moved on the table with a spiral path, which includes the movement of the x-ray tube. The rate of table movement during the scan is related to the speed of data acquisition defined by the concept of pitch, so a high or low pitch can be defined and controlled by the main computer of the CT system.

In addition, other important requirements apply. The table needs to be absolutely transparent to x-rays in the sliding part which is inserted inside the gantry. It must have comfortable contours for the patient and be easy to clean. Also, it is necessary to have the ability to attach accessories to facilitate the positioning of the patient, such as head supports, arm supports, knee pads and all kinds of bands for compression and security, and the possibility for conducting technical quality measurements, using phantoms and measuring instruments. Finally, all tables must have numerical values for selected indicators (such as height and travel distance) that are easily visible to the operator.

18.4 The gantry

The gantry is a fundamental element of a CT system [2]. It contains the initial part of the whole process of exploration, the tube and radiological detectors receiving radiation not absorbed by the patient. Therefore, its construction and reliability thereof will depend on compliance with the technical requirements of a device: picture quality, short reconstruction times and a low dose for the patient and others present.

The gantry contains a sensitive mechanical system that allows the harmonic and synchronized movement of the x-ray tube relative to the detector according the system used by the manufacturer. Some companies use a belt drive system to move the rotational part over the stationary part of the gantry. Others use a magnetic system of coils installed on one side and permanent magnets on the other side (these are the stationary and rotating drums, respectively) applying the principle of magnetic rejection and attraction controlled by varying the frequency and voltage on the coils from the control panel.

The gantry must contain a number of basic elements, namely: the x-ray tube, with the filters and the respective collimator, also the x-ray generator, detectors and the conversion system from analog to digital signals, all of which must be properly balanced. The entire assembly must be housed inside the gantry.

In addition to the function of allowing the rotation of the tube and the collection of information by the detectors, the gantry must have axial and angled tilting motions, and obviously have an adequate opening to receive any type of patient, even if they are obese. Figure 18.2 is a diagram of the contents of a gantry, which shows the group of detectors, the photomultiplier tubes and the electronic components comprising the data acquisition system. These are all integrated into a

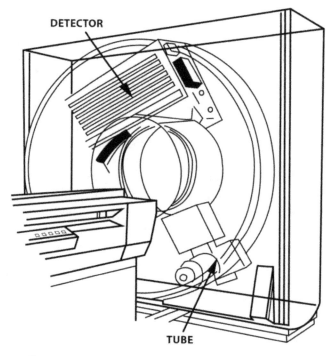

Figure 18.2. Gantry showing the detector array and the tube.

container located next to the central opening of the gantry block, at the opposite end to the x-ray tube. Synchronous rotation of both parts is only possible if there is a common mechanical support moving curved rails [3] which also allows the tilting movement.

The requirements for the gantry are also rigid in terms of the accuracy of its parameters, in particular in relation to the distance between the tube and the iso-center (the center of the opening of the patient location) of the gantry, as well as the distance between the iso-center and the detector. As in conventional radiography, the relationship established between the distances from the tube to the scanned object and thence to the detector (which in this case replaces the radiographic film) is important. The resulting magnification must satisfy the tradeoff between increased resolution and the need for more detectors. Thus proper accommodation of all the elements inside the gantry should be achieved to meet this requirement.

As shown in figure 18.3, if we increase the distance between the object and the detectors, a magnification exists which gives a better resolution, but as the object is located in a fixed position, such as the gantry iso-center, magnification can only be obtained if the tube approaches the patient, thus forcing open the range of radiation to cover the entire field of view (FOV). This means having as many detectors as possible; if not, some signal will be lost at the extremes of an arc detector. In the gantry other important concepts are determined, such as the scan speed and patient dose.

Technical Fundamentals of Radiology and CT

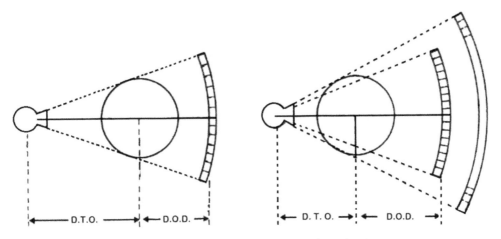

Figure 18.3. Different distances between tube and patient.

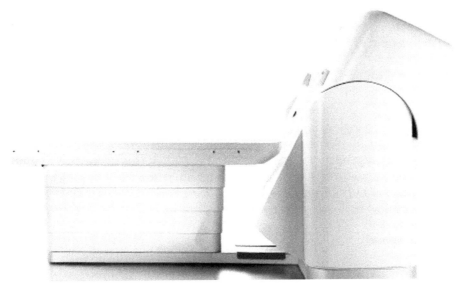

Figure 18.4. Gantry angulation. Courtesy of Koninklijke Philips N. V.

18.5 Requirements for the gantry

The gantry must be within the basic parameters in terms of distances, dimensions, speeds, etc. The main requirements are:
- The distance between the tube and the detector must be 1100 mm ± 10%. Some manufacturers use a tube–center distance of 630 mm and a detector distance of 470 mm to the iso-center. Other devices use a tube–iso-center distance of 780 mm and a 320 mm iso-center–detector distance.
- The gantry angle (tilt), should have an interval between ±20° and ±25°. The accuracy of the gantry tilt should be at least ±0.5°, some have an accuracy of 0.25° (see figure 18.4).

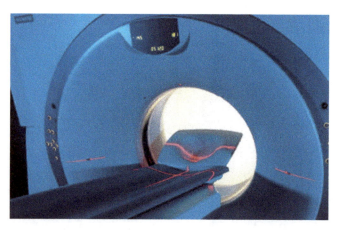

Figure 18.5. Laser lights for positioning. Courtesy of Siemens.

- The rotation of the tube with the detector system must be at least 360° for full exploration, and 210° for partial exploration
- The opening of the gantry must be in the range of 50–75 cm.

Other requirements related to the mechanical gantry are as follows. The rotation should be smooth and without vibrations. There should be several selectable rotation speeds (at least three) and an indication system if the patient is in contact with the gantry. Also, a locking system is necessary to prevent activation of the table or gantry tilt when the system is in rotation. The gantry must possess lateral and vertical lights for alignment when positioning the patient (see figure 18.5). Gantries also have a built-in audio system to enable communication with the patient in order to give instructions and ask questions during the examination [4]. Finally all kinds of gantries must allow easy access to the interior for maintenance and adjustments.

18.6 Scan speed

If the exploration is faster, the device is more efficient in terms of the number of patients it can study and its capacity to explore moving organs such as the heart. At the same time it minimizes the artifacts produced by involuntary movements of the patient. It is therefore intended that the rotation will be as fast as possible. This is achieved with excellent mechanical and electrical design: by an order from the operator, the tube assembly begins to accelerate, so that in less than a second it must be rotating at a constant speed and accuracy. After which the system gradually stops, arresting all movement in one second. Radiation is emitted only during the time when the system is rotating at a constant speed, during the 360° scan. As these turns are repeated thousands of times a year, very strict technology and design are required to maintain system reliability.

18.7 Radiation dose to the patient

The less time the patient is irradiated, the less dangerous is the study, so that a device must have the ability to obtain images with the lowest possible dose. Therefore, a short scan time and the emission of radiation in pulses are used. A permanent voltage value is applied to the tube, but there is a negatively polarized grid for controlling the radiation which prevents the electrons impacting on the rotary anode and producing radiation. For example, in the case of a scan that takes 4.8 s, 288 pulses are applied at intervals of 1/60 s, in the case of a scan of 9.6 s, 576 pulses are generated. With each pulse, the tube emits x-rays for a very short period (between 1 and 3.3 ms). Thus, the values of the control pulse duration, the number of pulses and the current chosen by the operator, are the factors that determine the dose on the patients. The most recent devices have software protocols that automatically select the optimal settings for each type of study.

18.8 Collimators and filters

In the gantry also we have the collimators and filters for compensation. The collimator serves to define the geometry of the radiation; in the case of fan systems one must determine the fan angle (between 30° and 50°) and the slit collimator to determine the thickness of the circular sector forming the fan (see figure 18.6).

The radiation beam must be filtered, so filters in some devices are selectable, with the function of reducing the radiation energies that do not contribute to image formation but are absorbed by the patient (see figure 18.7). Moreover, compensating filters are included in order to reduce the dynamic level of the analog–digital converters (located behind the detectors) and are responsible for converting the received signal into manageable data for the computer. The dynamic level of the narrowest converters requires a more sophisticated electronics system, but this effort is recommended, depending on the image quality required.

In any case it must be remembered that the problems caused by the broad spectrum of radiation are not resolved by only the filtering described. We must use a combination of means (hardware and software), and mathematical correction to compensate for the effects of the failure of obtaining monochromatic radiation. Another problem is the effect of radiation hardening, which produces deformation on images; the object studied appears less dense than the actual radiation compared

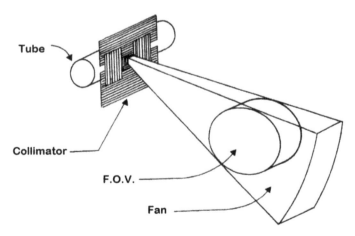

Figure 18.6. Function of a collimator.

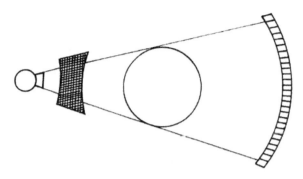

Figure 18.7. Radiation compensation of filters.

with monochromatic radiation (the ideal). Finally, it should be noted that there are two filters, one for the head and one for the body that the computer automatically inserts in most systems.

18.9 The radiation generator and control system

The CT radiation generating system consists almost exclusively of a special radiographic tube, a computerized high frequency generator and the electronic linkage with the computer to perform the irradiation in harmony with the chosen procedure [5].

18.9.1 The x-ray tube

The x-ray tube used in CT is special and must meet the following basic requirements:
- A rotating anode, grid controlled with a heat storage capacity of at least 700 000 caloric units (some tubes have more than 2.5 million HU).
- The metal housing must have at least 2 million HU and be protected against radiation leakage and mechanical shock.
- The tube should have a focal point of 1.2 mm (or less).
- Heat dissipation must be at least 150 000 BTU min^{-1}.
- The tube should have a capacity of maximum instantaneous load of 60 kW at 120 kVp.
- The cooling system must be based on oil circulation.
- The tube must have an adequate collimation range for the definition of a fan beam and also use pre-collimation in order to protect the patient through the best possible use of the dose.

18.9.2 The x-ray generators

Although many manufacturers initially used conventional radiological generators, the trend has become to build generators specially dedicated for maximum utilization of the system. The generator must meet, at least, the following requirements:
- A maximum voltage of 120 kVp.
- A large scale of tube current, from 50–500 mA.
- An automatic compensation of fluctuations in the network and a stabilization system for maximum high voltage accuracy.

– Computerized synchronization of the whole system [6] so that it works with all scanning mechanisms and allows the possibility of preventing overload of the tube, also indicating the process of emission of radiation in acoustic and visual forms.

18.10 The detection and processing system

The detection and processing system consists of two basic parts, the detectors and other components suitable for the most efficient use of radiation [7]. One of the most important components of any device is the set of sensors used to collect the radiation that passes through the patient, initiating the data acquisition involving a string of components, which ends with the image on the screen. Different types of detectors are used in CT, some based on ionized gases but the majority are semiconductor crystals. Table 18.1 shows the different types of detectors used in commercial CT scanners.

The main purpose of all types of detectors is to convert x-ray energy into electrical energy that can be manipulated by the computer. In the case of semiconductor detectors, the interaction of x-rays with the crystal structure of the semiconductor releases energy as a photon of visible light, so solid-state detectors require a photomultiplier tube to converting this signal of light into electrical output.

The most commonly used gas detector is the xenon detector, which works at low pressure and allows the conversion of the energy of the x-rays into gas ionization, i.e. when radiation beams are incident with the atomic structure of the gas molecules, free electrons are collected by an electrode which generates a voltage on a resistor in proportion to the amount of radiation received. There are also cesium iodide detectors (CsI), which have the unique quality of directly releasing electrons when they receive x-rays, so this type of detector does not require a photomultiplier.

The manufacturers of the various devices on the market argue for the advantages of their respective types of detector. In the early days of CT technique there was a marked difference between competitors. Now the main conflict is among the most used systems, sodium iodide detectors and xenon detectors, both of which have advantages and disadvantages.

The main advantage of crystal detectors is the number of elements that can be accommodated in the arc detector. Another important advantage is the high ratio of output to input—the electrical signal related to the received photons. This concept is known as the conversion factor, which in solid-state systems and amplifiers can reach 95%, while the conversion factor of gas detector systems has only reached 60%.

Table 18.1. The different types of detector used in commercial CT scanners.

Detector type	Formula
Calcium tungstate crystal	$CdWO_4$
Sodium iodide crystal	NaI
Calcium fluoride crystal	CaF_2
Bismuth germanate crystal	BGO
Cesium iodide crystal	CsI
Xenon (gas)	Xe

However, gas detectors, in particular xenon, have significant advantages, so they have remained a key component of the devices of some manufacturers over the decades. One of the most significant characteristics of gas detectors is the fact that the gas is held in a closed chamber. This keeps the gas uniformly distributed at a certain pressure, providing long-term stability, and making the gas insensitive to the effects of temperature and humidity. A particular advantage is the uniform response of all the compartments that constitute the detector. These cells are formed with channels or plates of tungsten on a ceramic base, as shown in figure 18.8.

In the input of the detector there is a thin aluminum window, facing the x-rays, and each of the plates is connected to a uniform voltage of 500 V. Whenever x-rays impact the detector ionization is produced, so that positive ions of xenon are collected by the middle plate between each cell, as shown in figure 18.9. To make a

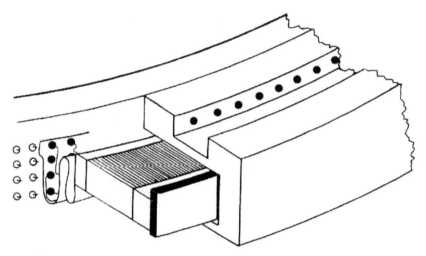

Figure 18.8. The structure of a xenon detector. Courtesy of General Electric.

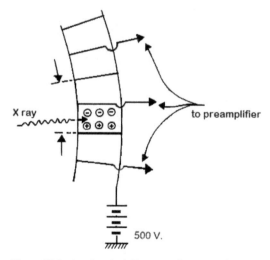

Figure 18.9. An electrical diagram of a xenon detector.

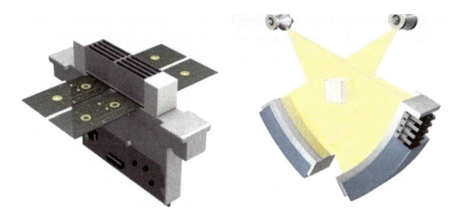

Figure 18.10. Solid-state detectors. Courtesy of Siemens.

proper comparison, one must know in detail the operation of the modes of collecting information with different types of detectors.

Crystal detectors are formed of a basic component, the crystal light radiation converter. These are made from the materials shown in table 18.1 and must have an electronic system for amplifying the weak light that the system generates. For this two fundamental structures can be used: a photomultiplier tube (as described above) which generates a growing flow of electrons with incident light, and a photodiode, which is a solid-state component and is also responsible for generating electrical signal from the light received. The two systems are compared in figure 18.10.

18.10.1 Properties of detectors

The conditions and requirements for the detector [8], will help to determine the convenience of using one detection method or another. A detector must have the following properties:
- Similar behavior for all cells.
- Parameters that remain constant regardless of temperature changes, moisture and aging effects.
- As many detectors as possible on the same cell surface.
- The minimum possible spacing between each cell.
- The greatest possible width of the cell with respect to the spacing between cells, this determines the concept known as the geometric efficiency of the detector. Higher is better, so if the geometric efficiency is high, the detector has better behavior as a whole.
- The highest possible discrimination range in the detector (not to be confused with the dynamic range of the analog–digital converter), which is the detector's ability to accept a broad level of intensities of x-ray output proportional to the input.
- A high ability to reject scattered radiation and accept only the primary radiation, this is achieved with good post-patient collimation.
- The lowest possible light inertia, i.e. not generating a light signal once radiation has ceased, this concept is known as afterglow.

- The highest possible value conversion factor, which is the ratio between the power output in relation to the light received.

With all the properties described above, we can compare the behavior of one detector type over another. In fulfilling these requirements we can see the significant advantages of xenon detectors over crystal detectors and some vice versa, namely:

- Every cell of a crystal detector is not exactly equal to its neighbors due to the natural differences arising from manufacturing processes, in the same way that two transistors of the same type are not exactly equal. For xenon detectors, each cell has metal walls that can be machined with great perfection and filled with a gas that is evenly distributed.
- Temperature and humidity changes have more obvious effects on systems of crystal detectors than those of gas. In fact, a sudden and drastic temperature change can cause breakage of the crystal. Also, components associated with crystal systems, for example the photomultiplier tubes, have a known degradation with age and photodiodes are also influenced by temperature.
- The number of cells can be increased in absolute terms in crystal detectors, but not in gas detectors. However, this parameter must be evaluated along with other elements, such as the spacing between cells (geometric efficiency) and fan radiation width. In any case this aspect of performance favors crystal detectors.
- Geometric efficiency is also better for gas detectors. If the separator sheet is closer and there is a wider face receiving the radiation, then there will be maximum utilization of incident radiation. However, if more detectors are located in the same length, the face of each cell becomes narrower, reducing the geometric efficiency.
- The dynamic range of gas detectors is also much higher than that of the crystal semiconductors, primarily because the photomultiplier tubes or diodes reduce the total dynamic range.
- Related to the rejection of scattered radiation, gas detectors use tungsten separating sheets as an anti-scatter grid acting as a collimator post-patient. Collimator leaves were added to crystal detectors with greater technical complexity to perform the same function, preventing overlap of the partitions between cells.
- The conversion factor is an important advantage of crystal detectors over gas detectors.
- Light inertia or afterglow exists only in crystal detectors and is their major disadvantage. Comparing the disadvantages and advantages, crystal detectors could compete very well with gas if they did not have the problem of afterglow.

Other factors related to the necessity of using photodiodes or photomultipliers introduce disadvantages for crystal detectors. Photomultipliers also degrade with age and have the disadvantage that slight changes in the power supply change their gain severely. As automatic stabilization circuits are required to constantly make adjustments, the total volume of the detector assembly is increased. Also, the system must rotate within the gantry, which means that it can be affected by the gantry's mechanical reliability.

Photodiodes have the drawback of a weak output signal, requiring high amplification, which introduces noise into the system, in addition to being affected by temperature. However, mounting the detectors with the photodiodes makes the gantry lighter and more reliable.

Today CT devices use a new type of super-detector, which combines the advantages of both systems. It has significantly low light inertia, high energy conversion and a small volume, is indifferent to temperature and humidity changes, has a uniform response in all cells, very good geometric efficiency and a high number of cells. Although the manufacturer does not provide technical details, protecting the confidentiality of its technology, it is known that the system is most likely based on solid-state detectors.

18.11 Geometric efficiency

We can measure numerically how much of the emitted radiation can be effectively received by the detector; this is the geometric efficiency. Figure 18.11 shows how certain rays are collected by each detector cell and how others fall into the spaces between the cells without producing useful information, which defines the relationship between openness and spacing.

A numerical example of evaluating the geometric efficiency of a detector is now presented, assuming that the value of the detector opening is 3 mm and the spacing between detectors is 4 mm. Then the ratio of geometric efficiency is:

$$GE = opening/spacing$$
$$GE = 3/4 = 0.86 = 86\%.$$

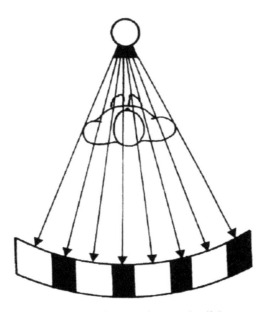

Figure 18.11. A diagram of geometric efficiency.

Technical Fundamentals of Radiology and CT

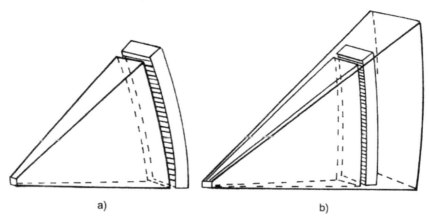

Figure 18.12. (a) High efficiency and (b) low efficiency of the fan beam.

This concept allows a numerical assessment of the quality of collimation of the fan beam in relation to the geometry of the detector, so that it can determine how much of the radiation generated traverses the patient producing useful information in a detector and how much is missed. The efficiency of the fan beam is measured by relating the detector width relative to the width of the fan of radiation. A comparison of two different radiation fans is shown in figure 18.12, one exactly matches the width of the detector (z-axis, relative to the patient), and the other has a greater range than the width of the detector, so that some information is lost, having been irradiated to the patient.

If a detector has a width of 1.5 cm and the collimated range has the same width, then:

$$\text{FWE} = \text{width of detector/width of fan}$$
$$\text{FWE} = 1.5/1.5 = 1 = 100\%.$$

In a second case, the fan has a width of 3 cm:

$$\text{FWE} = 1.5/3 = 0.5 = 50\%.$$

18.12 Conversion factor

As the conversion factor actually measures a gain of light, it is interesting to determine how much of the received radiation is converted into a useful electrical signal. The measured output signal, provided by each incident photon, translates to a conversion factor of 95% in the case of crystal detectors and only 60% for gas detectors (see figure 18.13).

18.13 Total dose efficiency

The concept of dose efficiency determines how much of the emitted radiation is usefully utilized in forming the image [9], and its numerical value is the result of the

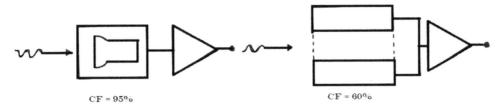

Figure 18.13. The conversion factors of a crystal detector and a gas detector.

factors described above. Thus dose efficiency is the product of geometrical dose efficiency (GE), fan width efficiency (FWE) and the photon conversion (PC) factor:

$$TDE = GE \times FWE \times PC.$$

Applying the numerical values used in the previous examples, a detector may have a total dose efficiency of:

$$TDE = 86\% \times 50\% \times 60\%$$
$$TDE = 0.86 \times 0.50 \times 0.60$$
$$TDE = 0.25 = 25\%.$$

The results indicate in which direction to work for the highest efficiency or the best use of the emitted radiation and thus quantifies, through objective measurements, the quality of the device related to the detectors, a key component of any CT system.

18.14 Requirements for detection

With all the data discussed in this chapter, it is possible to summarize the basic specifications [10] required for a detector system:
- The detector assembly should have no fewer than 520 cells and use a conversion system of photon energy into electrical energy. If the assembly has this many cells, at least 510 cells should be so-called patient detectors and 10 cells should be reference detectors. Some CT models far exceed these numbers, with 742 patient detector cells and 12 reference cells
- The detector must have a maximum spacing of 1.2 mm between cells.
- The shape of the detector and its structure must be such as to provide an angle smaller than 7° for the incidence of x-rays, so as to minimize scattered radiation.
- The geometric shape of the detector assembly must be such that the number of cells involved in receiving radiation, at any time, is no smaller than the following percentages:
  - 42% of the body must have 100% of the available cells.
  - A 35 cm body should have 50% of available cells.
  - 25 cm of the head must have 50% of available cells.
- The reference detectors should remain within the scanning radiation beam at all times.

18.15 The data acquisition system

The data acquisition system is defined as the set of electronic circuits that takes the electrical signal generated by the detector, turns it into a digital signal from analog values and delivers it to the computer that forms an image. The system must collect and sample the data at a rate at least equal to that of the network, i.e. 50 Hz or 60 Hz, and all data must be converted and transmitted to the computer within 20 ms or 16.7 ms, respectively. Some of the latest technology is able to handle 736 channels at a sampling frequency of 984 Hz and enter data into the computer in less than 1 ms. The effective range of analog–digital conversion is required to be at least 250 000–1. The best systems have a conversion range of more than 1 000 000–1.

Moreover, the electronics of the system must also be conditioned to carry out detector calibration using the reference detectors. Every system needs at least ten reference detectors. This set of detectors must be synchronized so that the calibration check takes place at least 200 times during a 5 s scan. This allows one to determine whether a single element or detector cell is defective.

The data acquisition system must be highly reliable and above all must have high precision and accuracy in handling information from the detector. Amplification must introduce the least possible noise, and analog–digital conversion must be complete and the dynamic range adequate in order not to lose information by saturation.

The dynamic range of the analog–digital converter [11] is the number of levels of each conversion step and the size of each step or stage of conversion. This determines the contrast resolution, i.e. the ability to detect small differences in the absorption of radiation in the tissue. If the steps have a difference greater than the size of the absorption detected, information is lost in the process of analog–digital conversion.

Figure 18.14 shows a simplified schematic of the process of analog–digital conversion. Numerical values are assigned to the size of the analog signal, and from there these numerical amplitudes are plotted, obtaining an approximate replica of the original signal. Obviously, the closer together the values are taken, the more similar the plot will look to the original.

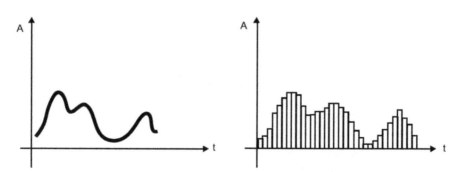

Figure 18.14. Analog–digital conversion.

Technical Fundamentals of Radiology and CT

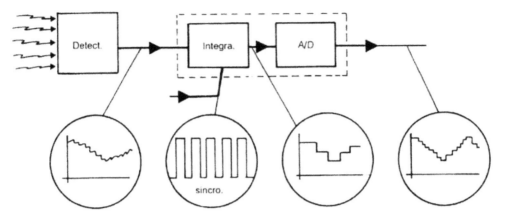

Figure 18.15. An outline diagram of a data acquisition system.

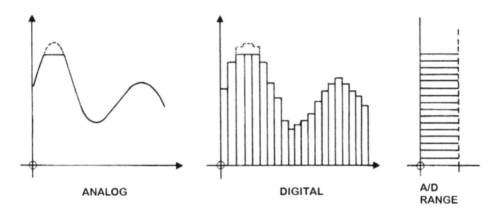

Figure 18.16. Assessment of dynamic range.

The advantages of converting a signal from analog to digital are primarily due to the fact that the numerical values of the amplitude expressed in binary values can be handled easily by computers [12] and the fact that this process has high immunity to noise, so that no deformations are subsequently introduced in image formation. Together with the signals generated by the detector that are to be converted to digital, positioning or timing pulses are used, relating to the successive measurement positions taken by the gantry. This is shown in figure 18.15. In figure 18.16 a conversion process is shown where we have insufficient dynamic range and the original signal is not properly recovered by the saturation of the converter, which cuts off part of the higher amplitude.

18.16 The formation of the image in the computer

From the digitized signal values, which are sometimes accumulated in a buffer, the host computer does all the work of image formation. It performs the functions of back-projection through logarithms and further convolution of the measurements,

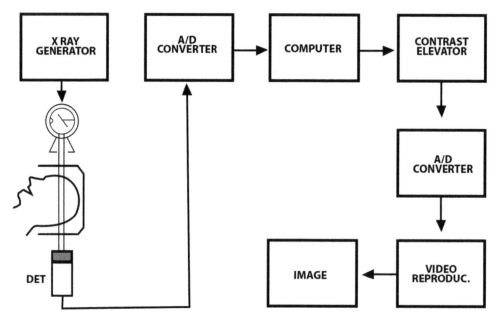

Figure 18.17. A block diagram of the measurement process. Courtesy of Siemens.

the allotment of grayscale values analog–digital conversion, and finally displays the image on a monitor, in black and white or in color.

Figure 18.17 shows a general block diagram of a processor device model manufactured by Siemens. Here we can see the key components of this configuration. Different manufacturers can use similar concepts in other configurations to achieve the same functions. Since this book is not intended to delve into the strictly computational aspects of CT, we will briefly explain these blocks of functions that are realizable by different methods.

The process of image formation involves the use of computers in various roles [13]. First the development of the absorption coefficient matrix, according to the concept explained in previous chapters, then from there assigning the different density values. In the conversion into grayscale, the Hounsfield scale is used. The values obtained are stored in a memory, wherefrom all the digital values are extracted line-by-line, to be handled by the adjustable window that allows the image to be represented at a level adapted to the eye of the observer.

The next step is to form an adequate image for display on the monitor in accordance with TV patterns. The information is read line-by-line from the memory array at the TV rate. The height of the TV image on the monitor is given by the number of scan lines of the video, and the width of each pixel on the screen is given by the length of reading time of each element of the array. Then the analog–digital converter transforms, also line-by-line on the matrix, all values found in the analog values that will form the combined signal, including the TV sync pulses which determine the classical standard signal that is sufficient to be applicable on any professional monitor or VCR.

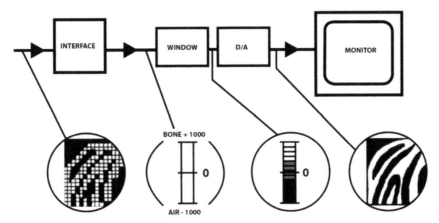

Figure 18.18. Forming video signal from the matrix.

This TV signal is presented with a polarity such that it allows us to see the whitest dense tissue (bone) and soft tissues with a darker tone, as seen on conventional radiographs. Figure 18.18 shows a schematic block diagram of the process of transformation from the array of pixels to the video signal representation of the same matrix.

The entire process chain [14] must include all the circuitry required for the formation of data relating to the process and the patient on the same image on the monitor, i.e. technical information, data exploration, patient data and institution data, etc. Alongside this, in the most complete devices, are included all the elements of hardware needed to perform various procedures [15] such as: sagittal or coronal reconstructions, dynamic sequence of images, extensions and zoom, modifications of formats, combining images, energy level changes, calibrated distances between selected points, evaluation of the region of interest, and so on. Figure 18.19 shown a more complete description of the steps required to form images from the digitized values collected at earlier stages.

All CT system image processors must have a main computer for data processing (the data processing subsystem) with a minimum capacity of 10 GB, 16-bit word parity checking and the possibility of expansion through additional boards. Some devices have a main memory of 120 GB.

18.17 Requirements for data collection and recreation

The data processing part of the system has some important requirements for hardware [15, 16], such as:
- A special purpose array processor with a floating point system.
- A microprocessor-based CPU.
- A word format with at least a 32 bit processor (array processor) for the floating point system.
- The processor for display images must meet the following specifications:
  - A matrix display of at least 512 × 512 by 12 bits to the level of −1024 to +3071 of the CT numbers.

- At least three separate planes for graphics memory overlay for annotations or additional images of at least 512 × 512.
- Two planes of independent memory for characters.
- A processor for the window interval, independent of the central processor unit, to handle at least 14 discrete values or continuous variation of the window interval.
- The logical cursor must handle at least five modes, grid, circle (or ellipse), rectangle, horizontal line and vertical line variables, to ±180°.
- Sixteen levels of grayscale range to display the image so that adjustments can be made to the brightness and contrast in the video.
- Video output of 8 bits corresponding to 256 or more grayscale levels.
- A system of non-interlaced video, to prevent the presentation of the video image on the monitor with fluctuations (i.e. achieve a flicker-free image).
- The imaging system must have the pixel sizes per FOV as shown in table 18.2.

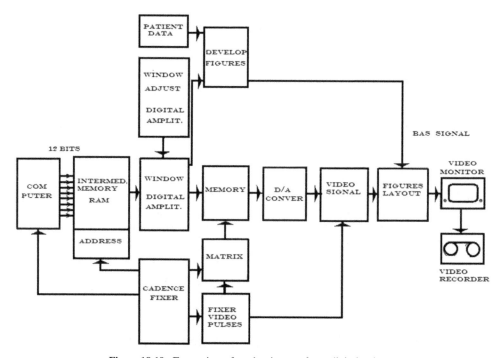

Figure 18.19. Formation of analog images from digital values.

Table 18.2. Required pixel sizes relative to FOV.

FOV	Pixel size
25 cm	0.8 mm
35 cm	1.1 mm
42 cm	1.3 mm

- The device should be able to make detailed reconstructions with pixel sizes as small as 0.13 mm with variable reconstruction centers.
- The system should have at least four selectable reconstruction algorithms: axial in standard or conventional modes, topogram plane [17] and detailed reconstruction of soft tissue or bone (bone detail).
- The system should enable the display of conventional images (axial) within 4 s of exploration and topogram planes 1 s after the scan.
- The system must be able to produce flashbacks in less than 45 s to soft tissue and bone detail.
- The system must have the ability to perform segmented reconstruction with more than three reconstructions for each scan data set.

18.18 Image display system and diagnosis

Everything discussed so far should be viewed by the device operator and physician as images on a screen. Thus the most appropriate image needs to be selected for viewing in order to decide whether to document the study or repeat it (which is fortunately not very common). The display system [18] generally consists of a console (see figures 18.20 and 18.21), which contains all the controls to perform the following functions:
- Direct the exploration, i.e. display all the values of the radiological generator, scanning speed, height and angle of the gantry, wide strata, anatomical exploration region, pitch selection, etc.
- Processing display images, i.e. the processing of the information obtained, its presentation on the screen, the choice of reconstruction algorithms and, in particular, the possibility of image manipulation with prompts,

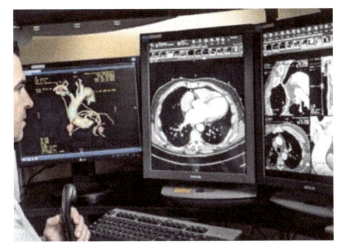

Figure 18.20. The appearance of a modern console. Courtesy of General Electric.

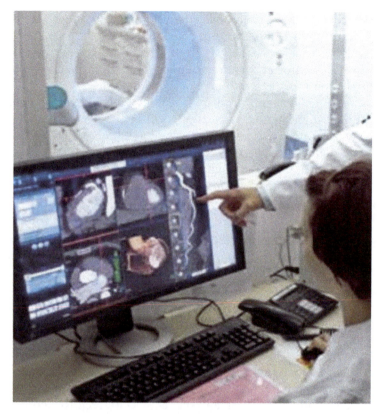

Figure 18.21. A diagnostic console. Courtesy of Siemens.

measurements, curves and histograms and other functions necessary to obtain the maximum information from the images.
- Sorting memory functions, file and image documentation in magnetic memory, disks, printers, x-ray film and so on.
- Notices and security mechanisms in the management of the complete installation, i.e. indication of excessive radiation, heating of the tube and gantry movements, and other prohibited processes.
- The possibility of aborting the scan for any emergency with the device or patient.
- Controlling audiovisual exchange with the patient.

In complete facilities an additional console is used, called the diagnostic console. This is used to assess previously obtained images while the device is working with another patient. The diagnostic console is usually connected to the common computer and thus can perform simultaneous operations, increasing system productivity.

Technical Fundamentals of Radiology and CT

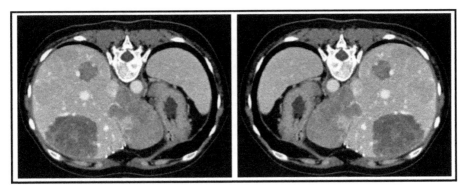

Figure 18.22. Inversion to the right and back to the left. Courtesy of Siemens.

18.19 Image manipulation

Most CT systems have the same functions relating to the presentation of images, and manufacturers compete to offer better options to their rivals. In general systems have the following features for the presentation of images [19]:

- Inversion from left–right and vice versa of the image on the screen.
- Reversing video from white–black or vice versa.
- Registration of alphanumeric data on the sides of the image, for which the system uses a suitable console keyboard.
- Defining one or more regions of interest (by the operator) consisting of a definable area, either by hand using a sphere (the track ball), a joystick or cursor keys in order to automatically measure the area defining an injury or disease, calculating the average absorption in the region, etc. The region of interest may have a circular or elliptical perimeter arbitrarily drawn by the operator.
- Automatic measurement of distances.
- Profiles for the absorption values in a region or between two points.
- The display of multiple images containing sequences of events or the development of a phenomenon, for example, the cardiac cycle or renal clearance.
- Presentation of the previous or next image that the operator wants to have on the screen.
- Indication of the scale of CT numbers (Hounsfield) in shades of gray on the side of the screen image.

In addition to the possibilities described above, the console must be able to perform other utilitarian functions, such as transferring data to an external memory or magnetic tape, even during scanning, operating a calibration program and system test functions, and displaying a list of patients and providing the possibility of removing, adding or altering the order thereof. Figures 18.22–18.30 show the application of these functions [20].

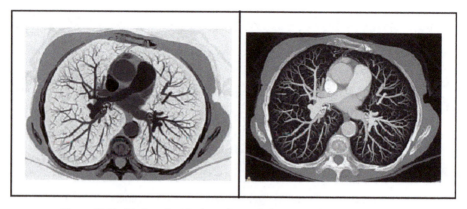

Figure 18.23. Black and white inversion and vice versa. Courtesy of Philips.

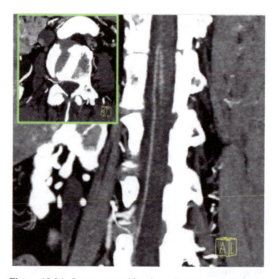

Figure 18.24. Image magnification. Courtesy of Siemens.

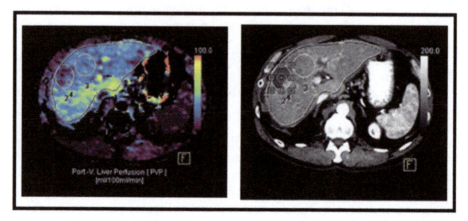

Figure 18.25. Regions of interest. Courtesy of Siemens.

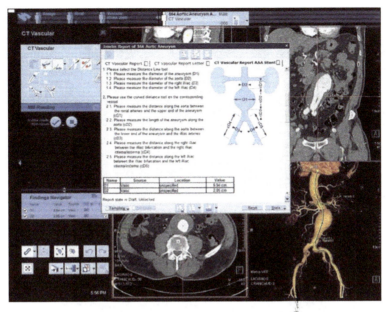

Figure 18.26. Measuring distances. Courtesy of Siemens.

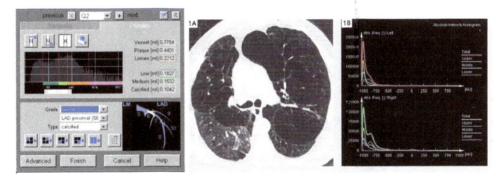

Figure 18.27. Histogram (left) and profile of CT numbers (right). Courtesy of Siemens.

18.20 Documentation of images

A pivotal function in CT devices is the process of proper documentation of images, either as snap-shots, images on paper, on x-ray film, etc, as the image on the screen is not sufficient for diagnostics. The device operator or radiologist examines the results and he/she must send the most accurate image possible with comments or a radiologist's report to the physician who ordered the examination.

Moreover, a key role is played by the archive of complete files with images and studies of each patient. This requires a peripheral device, endowed with an excellent memory capacity to store the maximum of possible studies. The components typically used to store images are:

 – Floppy discs.
 – Magnetic discs.
 – Magnetic tape.

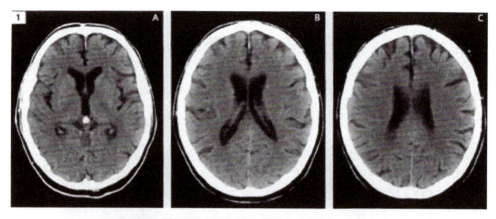

Figure 18.28. Several simultaneous images. Courtesy of Siemens.

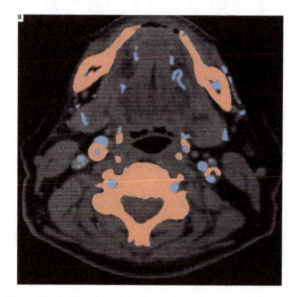

Figure 18.29. Lighting of similar regions. Courtesy of Siemens.

- Optical discs.
- Portable hard drives.
- Pen drives.

Magnetic tape can store up to 1000 CT images, while an optical disk cartridge can store up to a total of 30 000 images.

18.21 Recording devices

Other options to document studies (see figure 18.31) include:
- Polaroid cameras (obsolete).
- Multi-format cameras.

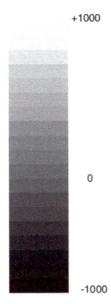

Figure 18.30. The grayscale used.

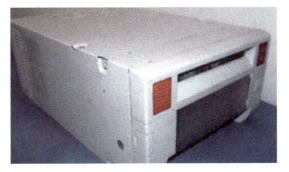

Figure 18.31. Video printer. Courtesy of Siemens.

- Photography cameras without a cassette.
- Video printers.
- Image scanners.

Multi-format cameras use common radiographic film contained in a cassette and, according to the selection of the operator, can record up to 12 images per film (see figure 18.32). These cameras also have the ability to select print speeds [21].

Video printers allow one to record directly from the video monitor signal. A reproduction of the image is printed on special paper. Although the quality and resolution of the image are not equivalent to those of a photograph, in most cases the images are sufficient in quality and the cost of using these devices is lower. Some

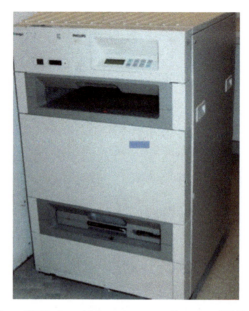

Figure 18.32. A multi-format camera. Courtesy of Philips.

appliances of Japanese manufacturers offer this device, which is also used in recording images of ultrasound studies.

References

[1] Ambrose J and Gooding M R 1976 EMI scan in the management of head injuries *Lancet* **1** 847
[2] Kuhler W 1978 CT scanning of the thorax *Xtract* **1** 12–8
[3] General Electric Medical Systems 1986 CT/T sagittal and coronal imaging *Product Data* B7900
[4] General Electric Medical Systems 1987 CT 9800 scanner system *Product Data* B7910JA
[5] Glujovsky M 1987 Tomograf SRT 1000: the power of x-rays *Sci. USSR* **32** 10–23
[6] Miller D, Dawes A and Cowie J 1985 Exploración por TAC de rutina del peñasco con reconstrucciones secundarias a partir de estratos de 1 mm de alta resolución *Electromédica* **1** 2–7
[7] General Electric Medical Systems 1986 CT/T independent diagnostic center *Product Data* B7800FA
[8] Zonneveld F and Vijverberg G 1984 The relationship between slice thickness and image quality in CT *Medicamundi* **29** 104–17
[9] DEGIEM 2012 Tomógrafo computarizado de 64 cortes *Especificaciones Técnicas Código* RX-15
[10] General Electric Medical Systems 1986 G.E. fast-scan CT: a whole new generation *Sales Data* ch 3
[11] General Electric Medical Systems 1987 System enhancement package *Product Data* B7805AA
[12] General Electric Medical Systems 1987 Dynamic scan capability *Product Data* B7815

[13] Alexander J and Krumme J 1988 Somatom plus: nuevas perspectivas en la tomografía computarizada *Electromédica* **2** 50–6

[14] General Electric Medical Systems CT/T 8000 scanner system *Product Data* B7840A

[15] General Electric Medical Systems 1986 Continuum CT/T: un progreso planificado *Catálogo de Venta*

[16] General Electric Medical Systems 1987 CT traveler (module IV) *Sales Data*

[17] General Electric Medical Systems 1987 CT/T optional diagnostic capability with scout-view localization system *Product Data* B7812

[18] General Electric Medical Systems 1989 CT/T technology continuum technical performance of the CT/T system *Technical Booklet*

[19] CENETEC 2009 Tomografía computarizada *Guía Tecnológica* No. 6 GMDN 39815

[20] Hitachi Medical Corporation CT-HF cranio-cervical computed tomography system *Spec Booklet*

[21] General Electric Medical Systems Quick-cam multiformat camera *Product Data* B79820GA

IOP Publishing

Technical Fundamentals of Radiology and CT

Guillermo Avendaño Cervantes

Chapter 19

Image reconstruction algorithms

19.1 Introduction

The most advanced devices are able use the data obtained to reconstruct images with different presentations [1]. Initially the studies were restricted to the conventional presentation of axial images, in which the full field of view (FOV) is displayed on the screen after completing the exploration and once the computer has completed the reconstruction.

Reconstruction algorithms exist to obtain different image presentations, which are intended for special studies or exploration of a specific region of interest. Other than the axial mode, other display modes are:

- Topogram or flat exploration.
- Details of soft tissue.
- Details of bone.
- Three-dimensional presentation.

There are also the serial scan, dynamic analysis (cine) and reconstruction in three dimensions [2]. All of these were initially optional, however, in modern devices their growing utility has made them practically mandatory.

19.2 Topograms

Unlike conventional axial CT scans, the topogram is a panoramic image of the region of interest, made with the same beam that is subsequently used for scanning. To obtain a topogram, unlike for a tomogram, the tube is fixed with the chosen detectors in a sagittal or frontal position, and the patient moves longitudinally (see figure 19.1). Every step of the longitudinal movement is irradiated and the information is collected. After a certain distance, e.g. 25 cm, the study stops and the computer proceeds to arrange the collected projections and form them into a flat image similar to conventional radiography, but with some advantages. The image is amenable to electronic manipulation of the window to specifically study any tissue or structure, and the image can be stored.

doi:10.1088/978-0-7503-1212-7ch19

Topograms were initially used only for localization purposes to explore a region, but are currently used for diagnosis, in particular in the region of the mediastinum (the lungs and chest bones). Topograms have a set of advantages for the radiologist, allowing the use of devices equipped with this application for comparative diagnosis. To use the topogram as a locator there is a cursor, usually marked by a white dashed line on the image plane, that the operator can move and place exactly in the region under study, and the computer moves the patient, placing them in the correct location to achieve the desired tomogram.

Some systems, in addition to displaying on the monitor a topogram previously obtained in the exploration, include in the tomographic image of the scanned region a small image of the topogram to help locate where the scan was performed. Figure 19.2 shows a frontal and a sagittal topogram on the screen.

Figure 19.3 shows three images, one each of the head, abdomen and pelvis, which include a reference topogram [3]. General Electric has registered the name 'Scoutview' for their topograms, while Phillips uses the name 'Scanogram'.

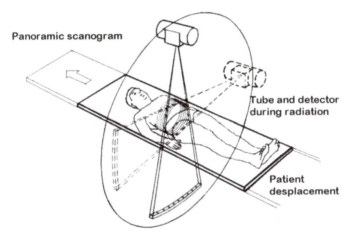

Figure 19.1. How to obtain a topogram. Courtesy of Siemens.

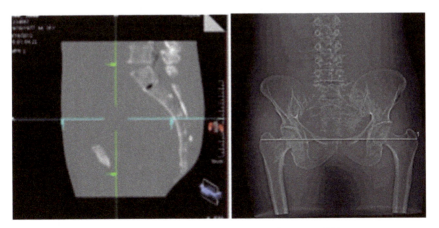

Figure 19.2. Frontal and sagittal topograms. Courtesy of Siemens.

(a)

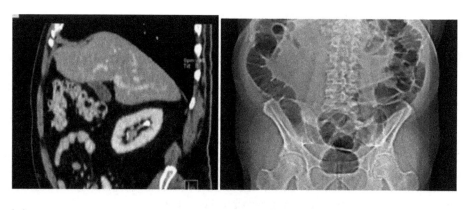

(b)

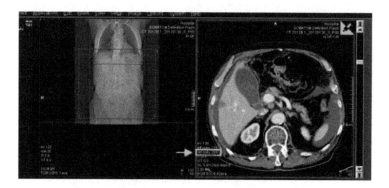

(c)

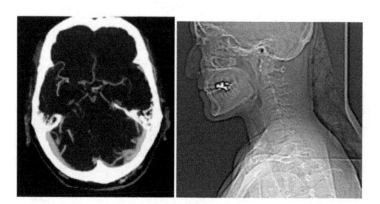

Figure 19.3. Topograms: (a) pelvis, (b) abdomen and (c) head. Courtesy of Siemens.

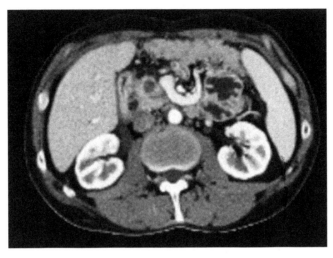

Figure 19.4. A detailed study of soft tissue. Courtesy of Siemens.

19.3 Algorithms for soft tissues and bone

When soft tissue studies [4] are performed, what matters is the fine detail of tissues for proper diagnosis. Organs such as the liver, pancreas, kidneys and bladder, among others, require a specialized algorithm to highlight both the spatial details and the density of the tissues. This is achieved through preset algorithms that consider a number of factors, such as the magnification of the region to study, the input values (mA, kV, mAs), the thickness of the layer and the scan duration, so that specific details of the relevant parts of the tissue can be observed. For example, in the abdominal study shown in figure 19.4, fine details are seen.

Algorithms are also necessary to perform detailed studies of certain delicate bones [5], such as spinal details in general and in particular studies of the delicate bones of the inner ear and the bones of the pelvis. To perform these studies, it is necessary to have a special algorithm which has, above all, a high discrimination of tissues and a high spatial resolution, in addition to being able to manipulate the window at the highest possible level. Another technical resource to reduce the contrast of the bone–soft tissue interface and thereby improve the clarity of the images of bone, is the automatic modification of the intensity of the monitor screen. This type of study also uses collimation, the layer width, the radiographic technique and generally the best possible use of the dose, in order to design an algorithm specialized for the study of bone tissue. Figure 19.5 shows the details of the bone structure of the inner ear, where you can see the cochlear detail, the facial nerve canal and other fine details.

19.4 Coronal and sagittal reconstruction

One of the most interesting applications of advanced software in contemporary devices is the possibility of generating coronal, sagittal and even oblique images, from previously obtained axial information. In this way we can visualize regions of the patient from other angles and positions without performing new explorations.

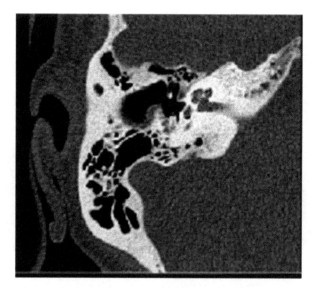

Figure 19.5. An image from a bone study. Courtesy of Siemens.

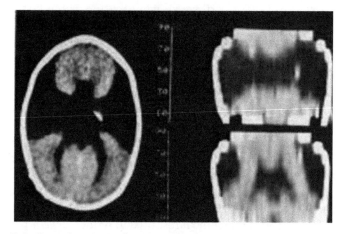

Figure 19.6. Coronal reconstruction of a cerebral hematoma. Courtesy of EMI images.

The clinical application of these new images is important in surgery, in pelvimetry (measurement of the pelvic bones) and in the measurement of bone in general, and in particular in mass evaluations of cysts, tumors, or any suspicious pathology in any structure that needs be to measured. Coronal or sagittal reconstructions, like the algorithms for soft tissue and bone, take a few extra seconds, allowing valuable diagnostic information to be obtained. Different devices use existing variable layer thicknesses and different numbers of layers to achieve reconstruction. The thickness of the layer plays a decisive role in the quality of the images obtained, both for conventional axial scans and for the sagittal or coronal reconstruction of a region.

Sagittal reconstruction [6] of the head is shown in figure 19.6, in which a cerebral hemorrhage is located with a conventional tomogram and then reconstructed from

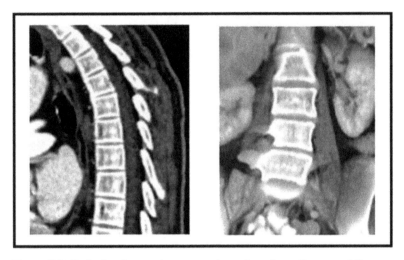

Figure 19.7. Sagittal and coronal reconstructions of vertebrae. Courtesy of Siemens.

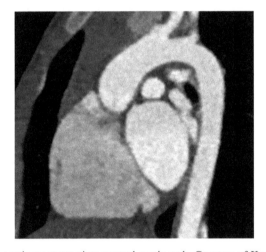

Figure 19.8. Oblique aortic reconstruction: normal aortic arch. Courtesy of Koninklijke Philips N.V.

the region defined by the white line of the study. The amount of bleeding can be evaluated by vertical sagittal reconstruction. These images were obtained with an old device (from three decades ago) manufactured by the company EMI. The images in figure 19.7, of sagittal and coronal reconstructions of vertebrae and the spinal canal, were produced using a CT device produced by Siemens, in the same period. Today we can expect to obtain significantly superior images. Using the same technique and appropriate software, oblique reconstructions of structures with difficult access and without having to move the gantry can be obtained. Figure 19.8 shows the oblique reconstruction of the aorta after taking a set of axial images of the region of the great vessels and heart.

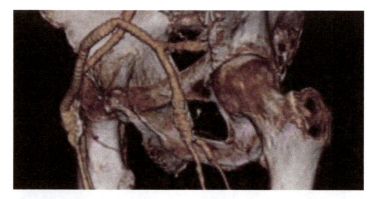

Figure 19.9. Selective three-dimensional reconstruction. Courtesy of Siemens.

19.5 Three-dimensional reconstruction

Three-dimensional reconstruction [7] is a powerful diagnostic and educational tool, and can be achieved through specialized high-capacity algorithms, which allow us to visualize the tissues of interest only, as shown in figure 19.9, where we see the articulation of the femoral head in the image excluding the rest of the tissues of the region.

References

[1] General Electric Medical Systems 1987 CT traveler (module IV) *Sales Data*
[2] General Electric Medical Systems Display enhancement package *Product Data* B7914DE
[3] General Electric Medical Systems CT/T optional diagnostic capability with scout-view localization system *Product Data* B7812
[4] Rienmulller R, Sommer B, Doppmann J and Schatzl M 1981 El topograma en el marco de la tomografía computarizada del mediastino *Electromédica* **2** 117–21
[5] Hulls A, Schulte W, Voigt K and Eirlich V 1983 Tomografía axial computarizada de la articulación temporomaxilar: nuevas posibilidades diagnósticas y primeros resultados clínicos *Electromédica* **1** 14–9
[6] General Electric Medical Systems CT/T Sagittal and coronal imaging *Product Data* B790ü
[7] Wallace M J *et al* 2008 Three-dimensional C-arm cone–beam CT: applications in the interventional suite *Vasc. Interven. Radiol* **19** 799

IOP Publishing

Technical Fundamentals of Radiology and CT

Guillermo Avendaño Cervantes

Chapter 20

Applications of CT

20.1 Introduction

The advantages of CT over conventional x-rays can be summarized as the utility of the images obtained for accurate, reliable and repeatable diagnosis, that can be made by both the radiologist and specialist requesting the examination. The tremendous technical complexity of designing and manufacturing CT devices is fully justified when a complex study delivers several images that make the diagnosis undisputed. Additionally, the latest sophistications allow the use of the entire arsenal of resources of hardware and software to complement and certify previous diagnostic assessments, with extensions, dynamic images, reconstructions, three-dimensional images, etc.

However, there is controversy regarding the potential development of applied technology [1] to provide even better results. Some experts claim that we are 'reaching the ceiling' of possibilities, and others believe that nuclear magnetic resonance imaging will replace CT. Currently, and for a long time in the future, this technology will probably remain the main tool in the diagnosis of various ailments and diseases.

To study the diagnostic applications of CT it is necessary to understand that the images that are obtained are essentially axial, so the radiologist should modify their somewhat conventional concepts about these images. He/she must become accustomed to looking at images with different criteria, in terms of anatomical dissections and not as x-rays of superimposed planes. Thus it is necessary to define the human body in accordance with its main anatomical planes and from them understand how cuts are made and what features they present.

20.2 Body planes

As shown in figure 20.1, the body is divided into three main anatomical planes:
- The sagittal plane.
- The coronal plane.
- The axial or transverse plane.

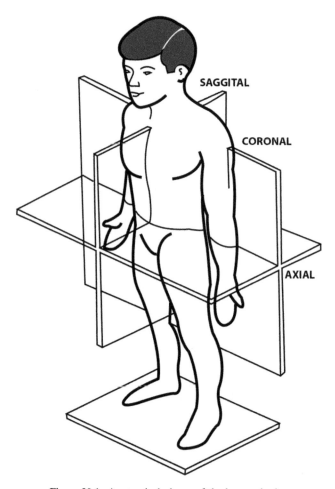

Figure 20.1. Anatomical planes of the human body.

The sagittal plane passes vertically through the body [2], dividing it into left and right. The coronal plane also passes vertically through the body separating it into front and back. The transverse or axial plane divides the body into two parts, upper and lower, and is situated perpendicular to the sagittal and coronal planes. This plane is the most interesting because the images obtained in CT are axial.

20.3 Directions

In addition to the body planes, it is necessary to determine the directions in which the anatomical reference [3] is made (see figure 20.2). These have the following possibilities:
- Medial and lateral.
- Posterior and anterior.
- Cranial and caudal.

Technical Fundamentals of Radiology and CT

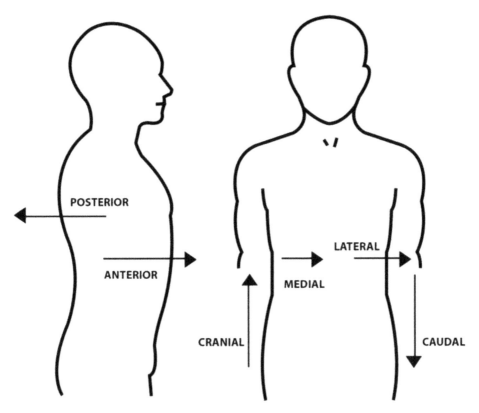

Figure 20.2. Anatomical reference directions.

The medial and lateral directions are opposite to each other, the medial being directed toward the mid-sagittal plane and the lateral from the mid-sagittal out of the body. The anterior and posterior directions are also opposite, anterior being directed towards the front of the body and posterior towards the back of the body. The cranial and caudal directions refer to shifts towards the head and feet, respectively.

20.4 Anatomical references

Since most studies of CT are performed on the head and trunk of the body, knowledge of anatomical references is required for studies [3]. Such references are external markings that relate to the internal organs, mainly contained in the cranial cavity, the thorax, the abdomen and pelvis (see figure 20.3).

The anatomical references [4] (numbered in accordance with figure 20.4) are:
1. The sternal notch.
2. The sternal xiphoid.
3. The navel.
4. The iliac crest.
5. Floating ribs.

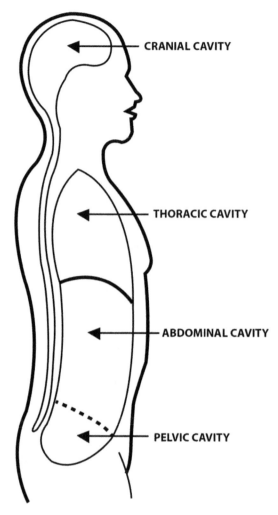

Figure 20.3. The main body cavities.

Figure 20.4 shows the anatomical references as well as the internal organs of the cavities of the trunk. These marks are used as the references necessary to guide tomographic studies.

To help in carrying out studies, CT systems have predefined protocols. These protocols automatically position the patient in relation to the references points at the push of a button. The table moves to place the patient in the requested position, which allows multiple scans or the study of various strata within a region defined by the references. Thus, if we want to perform a study of the liver, the patient will be positioned between the sternal xiphoid and the floating ribs, so the device will perform the requested scans in that region.

20.5 An axial view of anatomy

The main regions studied (the head, thorax, abdomen and pelvis) each have a characteristic shape that the radiologist interprets. According to the location and relationship of references, different images can be created, as shown in figure 20.5.

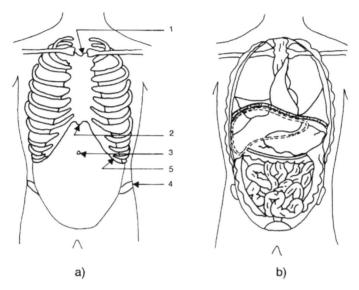

Figure 20.4. (a) Anatomical references and (b) internal organs.

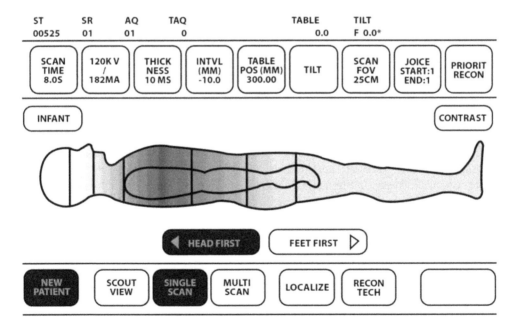

Figure 20.5. Automatic selection of areas of study.

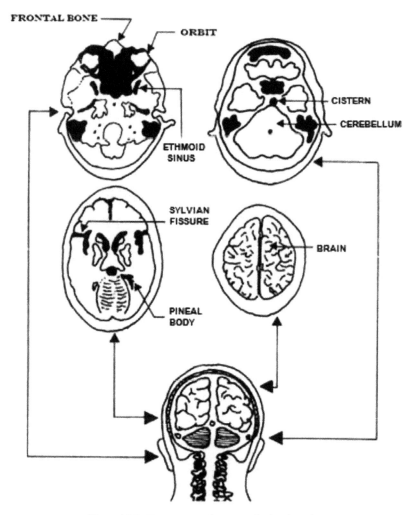

Figure 20.6. Four progressive cuts of a head study.

In the case of the organs of the head, such as the organs of sight and hearing, the external reference used is the back of the last vertebra (the atlas) and internal references are also used. Figure 20.6 shows a progressive scan which runs from the base of the skull to the top of the head down the middle of the ear.

In the first case the axis connecting the eye and the center of the ear canal is the reference, and the top left-hand image shows a section in which the lenses and optic nerve appear clearly visible, as do the ethmoid sinus and occipital bone. In the top right-hand image the temporal lobes, the cerebellum and the base of the fourth ventricle are visible. In the bottom left-hand image the head of the caudate nucleus, the Sylvian fissure, the interhemispheric fissure, the pineal body and the ventricles showing the lateral horns are visible. The bottom right-hand image has an almost unique view of the brain and the skull bones showing the interhemispheric fissure.

Studies of the trunk support many possibilities [5], with scans from the top of the thoracic cavity to the bottom of the pelvis, with a characteristic cut for each of the

Technical Fundamentals of Radiology and CT

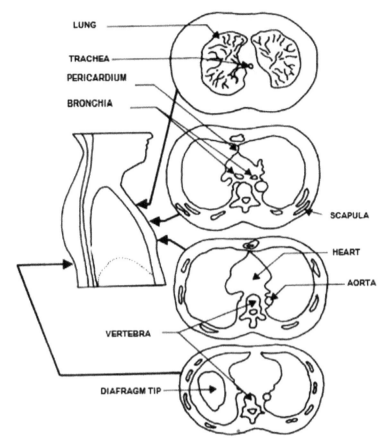

Figure 20.7. Four thoracic cavity cuts.

regions in which different bodies show a typical profile. Figure 20.7 shows four typical cuts of the thoracic cavity. The top image defines the window to observe the lung tissue in detail, although the bones and the heart do not have the same density, they are not visible by being outside the range of gray tones corresponding to the lungs; the central spot is the trachea. This image is located in the region of the upper mediastinum, below the junction of the two bronchial trunks in the trachea (the carina). The second image shows a section of the middle mediastinum level near the top, at the height of the sixth vertebra, so that we can see the characteristic shape of the scapula between the ribs and skin, and the bronchi in the middle with the heart in front. In the third image the descending aorta is clearly visible near the vertebrae [6], as is the cavity formed by the ribs and sternum, with the heart at the center and a lung at each side. The last image, taken at the end of the sternum (the xiphoid) shows a section of diaphragm muscle at the bottom of the lungs.

The most explored region statistically is the abdominal cavity, because there are many different studies of the liver, spleen, pancreas, kidneys, stomach, intestines, etc [7]. The typical and characteristic shapes of cuts made at different heights in the abdominal cavity are shown in figure 20.8. The top image is taken at the diaphragm level in a cut perpendicular to the eighth false rib and shows the liver, major vessels, aorta and

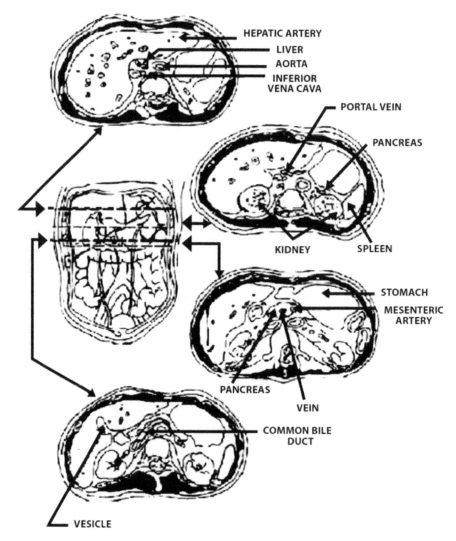

Figure 20.8. Four images of cuts in the abdominal cavity.

inferior vena cava, the medial part of the spleen, and of course the spine and rib cage. The second image is obtained at the penultimate rib and shows the top of the kidneys, the tail of the pancreas and the caudal part of the spleen. The third image (taken at the lowest level of the four) shows a cut passing through half the stomach (on the left side of the patient), while the right side shows the last lobe of the liver, the artery and the mesenteric vein (which are clearly visible in the middle), part of the duodenum on its downward curve, the left side of the heart (on the right in the image) and the upper aorta near the transverse colon. In the bottom image we can see the middle of the gallbladder through the liver. The common bile duct, the splenic vein and the caudal end of the spleen are clearly visible along with part of the duodenum below the liver. In this position we can see some vessels of the pancreatic duct.

Technical Fundamentals of Radiology and CT

A clear understanding of the configuration of the images in each of the regions is important, not only for the radiologist, but also for the radiology technician and engineer who work with the equipment. It is necessary to distinguish normal and pathological images from those presenting artifacts or deformations of electronic origin (the detectors and data acquisition) and those that may result from errors in the calculation of the values that make up the reconstructed image. We also have to always keep in mind that the window and its management can determine significant changes in the presentation of the image, accentuating some structures and virtually obliterating others. Therefore, the eye of the engineer needs to be accustomed to the classic form of CT images.

Figure 20.9 shows four characteristic cuts of the pelvic cavity. The top image shows the ilium (which is present throughout the pelvic region on the edge of the iliac crest) the fifth lumbar vertebra and, on both sides, the psoas muscles. The second

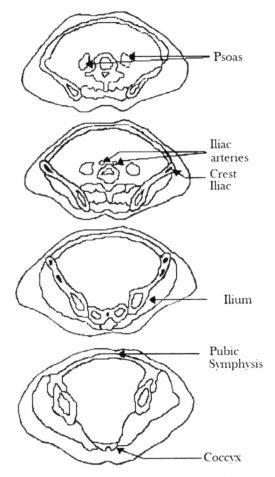

Figure 20.9. Four images of the pelvic cavity.

image clearly shows the iliac arteries, a cut through the iliac crest, the top of the sacrum and details of the sacroiliac joint. The third image shows the lower part of the ilium with the two rings that it forms. The bottom image shows the coccyx which is raised relative to the back of the pubic symphysis.

References

[1] Diejer N 1986 *Application of B&K Equipment to Diagnostic Ultrasound* (Naerum: Bruel and Kjaer)
[2] Jacob S W and Francone C Λ 1980 *Structure and Function in Man* (Philadelpia, PA: Saunders)
[3] Hanefee W 1988 Radiology the expanding fields *Hospimedica* **6** 11–3
[4] Metrevelli C 1987 *Practical Abdominal Ultrasound* (Oxford: Heinemann Medical)
[5] Desiré Ch Villeneuve F 1977 *Anatomía, Fisiología e Higiene* (Barcelona: Montaner y Simon)
[6] Kreel L and Osborn S 1976 Transverse axial tomography of the spinal column: a comparison of anatomical specimens with EMI scan appearances *Radiography* **42** 73
[7] General Electric Medical Systems 1986 GE fast-scan CT (anatomy) *Product Data*

IOP Publishing

Technical Fundamentals of Radiology and CT

Guillermo Avendaño Cervantes

Chapter 21

The most common CT studies

21.1 Introduction

Currently, the application of CT in every-day medical practice largely involves a set of routine diagnostic studies for the head and trunk. Assessments of trauma, scoliosis and pelvimetry are common. There are also some very specific types of extremity studies and other studies such the examination of pectus excavatum.

The first images obtained of the inside of the skull (figure 21.1) showing the lateral ventricles, were in themselves a great success [1], because the mere fact of determining their location and eventual displacement fully justified the advantages of CT compared to conventional radiography.

Figure 21.1 shows the classic matrix of the digital reconstruction, where the pixels are visible, which is characteristic of the first images obtained (in 1974). After this time, in the short term, it was possible to achieve better images using a specific computational device. The software continued to become more complex and increasingly efficient in improving the quality of images, and current images are now of such good quality that any doctor, even without specialized training or great diagnostic experience, can determine the class and even the boundaries of an injury or illness [2].

The use of filters, mathematical corrections and powerful algorithms that can work at high speeds and with large volumes of data is of immense value for the current images. These developments have been accompanied by significant advances in computing and radiographic hardware, which have led to spectacular results in current CT.

Figure 21.2 shows more modern images and emphasizes the great difference with respect to the first images obtained. Panel (a) is an early image, showing a normal brain with good tissue differentiation between gray and white matter, the ventricles are apparent. Panel (b) shows the soft tissues and details of bone, with the sinus cavities. Panel (c) images of cranial bones, with excellent details of the nasal bones, ears and eyes including the optic nerve. In panel (d) a case of meningioma is shown.

doi:10.1088/978-0-7503-1212-7ch21   21-1   © IOP Publishing Ltd 2016

Technical Fundamentals of Radiology and CT

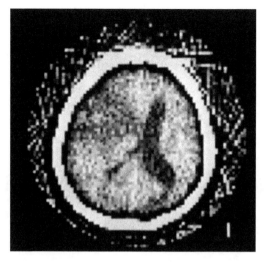

Figure 21.1. The first images of the inside of the skull with the Siretom system. Courtesy of Siemens.

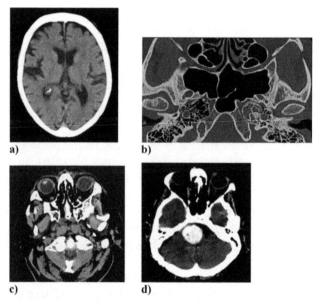

Figure 21.2. Improvements in images of the brain. Courtesy of Siemens.

21.2 Studies of the head

CT is currently used in the study of most diseases that require some intracranial knowledge, such as bleeding, obstruction and tumors of all kinds (astrocytomas, adenomas, neuromas, medullo-blastomas, craniopharyngiomas, meningiomas, lipomas process, chondromas, pineal tumors, adenomatous tumors, etc). CT is also suitable for studying the bones of the inner ear, the exploration of the petrous part of

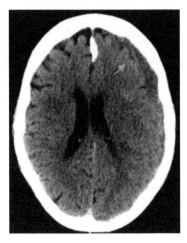

Figure 21.3. Cerebral bleeding. Courtesy of Siemens.

the temporal bone, including studies related to encephalic nerves and vessels [3]. CT is of fundamental importance in the diagnosis of all types of brain and head injuries, and strokes. Thus CT devices are diagnostic tools of primary importance in the emergency room of any hospital. The application of CT in studies of the bones of the head is useful, including in the study of the temporomandibular joint, which has become a revolutionary method that is demonstrably superior to dental radiology, including dental planigraphy.

The image in figure 21.3 shows a classic sign of pathology in the brain. An ischemic stroke appears with the expected gray tone deviated to white, which means an increase of absorption [4] and is explained by the presence of edema compression. In contrast, a cerebral infarction results in decreased absorption of x-ray radiation. Calcifications also have a tendency to appear as white, calcifications in intracranial regions are relatively easy to diagnose from images.

Figure 21.4 shows a case of severe calcification within the brain. Figure 21.5 shows a detailed view of the internal ear bones, numbered as follows: 20 = cochlear first spiral, 21 = cochlear second spiral and 22 = section of vestibulocochlear nerve in the cochlea.

The bones of the mouth related to chewing can be studied in detail using CT. Thus, arthropathy of the temporomandibular joint can be evaluated with significant advantages over other less accurate methods (see figure 21.6).

Studies of the spiral cochleae are of great importance, because before the advent of CT it was not possible to obtain significant details [5]. Currently it is possible to obtain information on both the medulla and the bone itself, apophysial details can be clearly seen and both the size and the shape of the spinous processes can be clearly delineated. Although studies related to the spinal canal were initially comparable to those obtained with myelography, they are currently of great diagnostic significance in cases of spinal stenosis or neurological masses. Figure 21.7 shows enlarged details of the spinal cord.

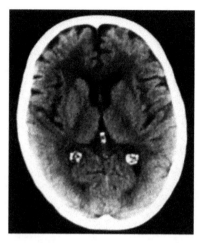

Figure 21.4. Cases of cerebral calcification. Courtesy of Siemens.

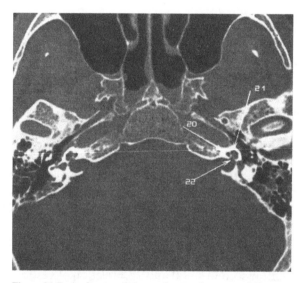

Figure 21.5. An image of the ear bones. Courtesy of Siemens.

21.3 Studies of the thorax

Within the thoracic cavity we can essentially perform studies [6] of the lungs, bronchi, major vessels, heart and, with quite remarkable success, women's breasts. Figure 21.8 shows (left side) a conventional mammogram where calcification is seen, which examined with CT (right side), is exposed so that can be better defined with a cursor and also enlarged with zoom. Figure 21.9 shows a tomograph of a female breast with a noticeable difference between the two breasts, having an extended mass clearly visible on the left side.

Lung studies are unique in requiring a very low window to view internal lung tissue, however the possibility of discrimination is lost in other tissues that appear as

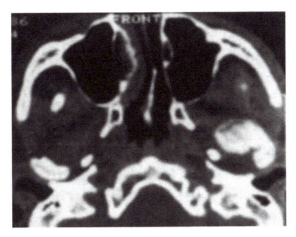

Figure 21.6. An image of the temporomandibular joint and condylar detail. Courtesy of Siemens.

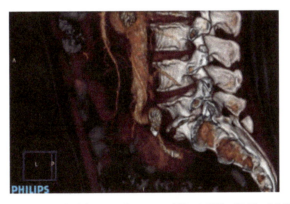

Figure 21.7. Spinal images. Courtesy of Koninklijke Philips N. V.

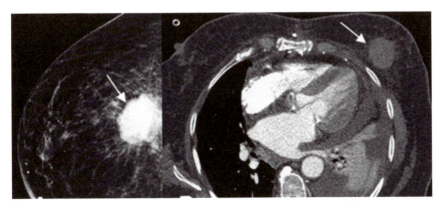

Figure 21.8. CT breast image showing calcification. Courtesy of Siemens.

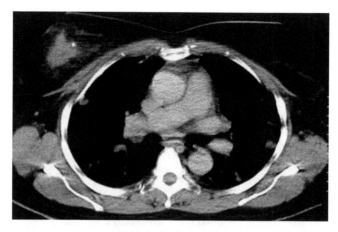

Figure 21.9. Breast CT.

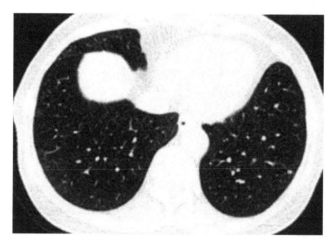

Figure 21.10. A pulmonary cancer. Courtesy of Siemens.

white or shades of gray close to white. Figure 21.10 shows the presence of an angioma.

In the case of professional diseases such as pneumoconiosis, asbestosis or silicosis, CT is also used successfully for accurate diagnosis [7]. Figure 21.11 shows a case of asbestosis, using a three-dimensional reconstruction of both lungs and color highlighting the lung regions most affected by the pathology.

21.4 Cardiac studies

Although the normal movement of the heart is considered a limitation on the quality of the images, due to the problem of artifacts produced by movement, valuable studies can be achieved by fulfilling some fundamental conditions:
- The device must have as short a scan time as possible to reduce image diffusion.

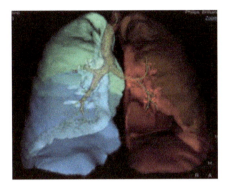

Figure 21.11. Image of asbestosis. Courtesy of Koninklijke Philips N. V.

- It is necessary to reduce other possible movements of the chest cavity, such as breathing, which should be sustained, if possible, with the patient's cooperation.
- The timing of the radiological shots needs to be synchronized with the electrocardiographic activity of the patient, so that the R wave of the EKG is the factor that governs the emission of radiation and the movement of the gantry.
- The devices needs to have a software discriminator for the resultant images, with a high index of artifact reduction [8], so that inappropriate images can be eliminated.

The need for heart tomograms, despite the drawbacks, is based on the fact that the resolution of CT can show, better than any other procedure, tissue changes in the heart muscle and also allows accurate delineation of the boundaries between the heart chambers. It is also of great physiological importance to study the dynamics through images displayed in succession (in the style of a film projection), showing the real-time operation of this vital organ. Furthermore, it is possible to use CT to dynamically assess the status of vascularization [9] before density measurements and after palliative or corrective cardiopulmonary surgery, which is not possible to achieve reliably using other diagnostic methods.

The diagnostic applications of CT in heart studies are highly significant, for example, studies of the dimensions of the chambers, particularly the relationship between them, measuring the thickness of the ventricular walls [10], both for diagnostic and scientific studies, and determination of injuries and wounds. Detecting ventricular septal defects and the identification of thrombi are very specific and delicate applications that can also be performed successfully, as well as infundibulum stenosis studies, studies during complex tetralogy, etc. The advantage of CT over ultrasound has been established in studies with both techniques, in which the deformations of chest and emphysema constitute between 10–15% of all the cases studied. A very important application of CT is the coronal, sagittal or oblique reconstruction of tomograms obtained in cases of aortocoronary bypass transplants. The images obtained allow tracking control in the progress of these common transplants.

Figure 21.12 shows structures in detail: rV and rA are the right ventricle and right atrium, Vc and Vp are the vena cava and pulmonary vein, and Aa and Ad are the ascending and descending aortas, respectively. The thin arrow shows the bypass to the right coronary artery and the thick arrow indicates the atrioventricular artery.

Figure 21.13 shows the case of a coronary transplant artery bypass [11]. In the left-hand panel the arrow points at the graft to the left anterior descending artery with the pulmonary artery (PA) of greater caliber. The right-hand panel shows the coronal reconstruction (made using with multiple images, as explained previously), wherein the arrow indicates the path of the proximal descending artery graft. The reconstruction shown is performed in the plane indicated by the line in the image on the left. VC is the superior vena cava, Ao the ascending aorta, LA the left atrium, DAo the descending aorta and LV the left ventricle.

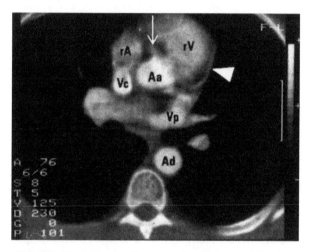

Figure 21.12. A coronary bypass study. Courtesy of Siemens.

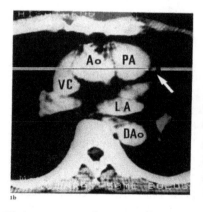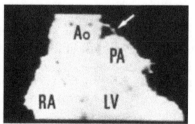

Figure 21.13. A tomogram of a coronary transplant artery bypass (left). Coronal reconstruction (right). Courtesy of Siemens.

A lot of studies are performed in the abdominal cavity. Organs such as the liver, spleen, kidneys and pancreas are routinely screened, yielding images that are fundamental to more accurate diagnoses and statistically provide a significant cost reduction compared to conventional studies, in terms of medical man hours and hospitalization time, almost to the level achieved with the use CT for head studies. The liver is one of the organs commonly examined, either to find cysts, tumors or metastases. Figure 21.14 shows a study with metastases presenting as tissues of darker shades of gray.

Pancreatic CT has proven to be highly accurate for the characterization and differentiation of masses with varied etiology, which were difficult to identify when this technology was first introduced. Figure 21.15 shows an abdominal scan with the pancreas in excellent detail.

In the abdominal region studies are also performed [12] on the intestines, using contrast media to highlight overlapping structures and to prevent the gases (as

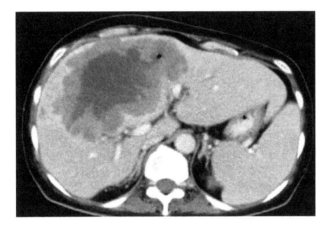

Figure 21.14. Liver metastases. Courtesy of Siemens.

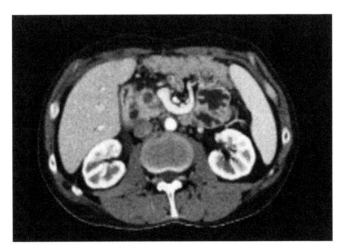

Figure 21.15. Abdominal image showing the pancreas in detail. Courtesy of Siemens.

occurs in conventional radiography) showing only dark spots (a low absorption of radiation).

Kidney studies are currently of great importance, not only for the anatomical visualization of the kidneys and the potential detection of tumors, cysts, vertebral lesions [13], etc, but also for the possibility of studying the physiological process of kidney excretion through mathematical manipulation of the time and density changes produced by tumors and other processes. This requires that the CT scanner performs a series of studies at high speed (serial studies), a function that is available in the best contemporary devices, and also requires the ability to perform calculations from images with specialized algorithms. It should be noted that quick scans and subsequent mathematical manipulation of the results are also applied in other case studies such as aneurysmal bone cysts, various tumors, thymomas, etc. The method proceeds through injecting a dye that produces a change in the absorption of radiation of the organ of interest as the series of scans is taken. Then the computer calculates and plots the change of Hounsfield numbers, both in the main feeding vessel, as in the case of a tumor, and defined by the region of interest selected by the operator [14].

In the control of kidney embolized tumors, a process that is virtually impossible from the angiographic point of view, CT is of great importance. Renal perfusion and its representation allow the observation of the tumors and their behavior in relation to the renal vein or inferior cava vein. CT is also an important application for controls during kidney transplants. Figure 21.16 shows the case of a transplant rejection; the graphics included on the screen simultaneously display the density–time relation of the transplanted kidney and the iliac artery, marked with I and II, in their respective regions of interest in the image. The graph shows the characteristic variation of the flow density in the iliac artery and on other side, with the curve of the transplanted kidney perfusion showing a plateau shape, a delay in the increase of the curve and the maintenance of a constant density. Thus the rejection condition is evident.

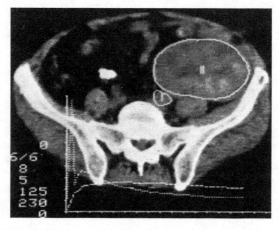

Figure 21.16. Kidney transplant rejection. Courtesy of Siemens.

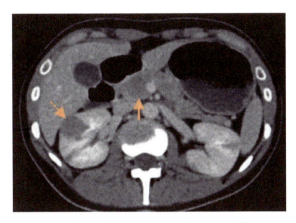

Figure 21.17. A visible lymphoma. Courtesy of Siemens.

Apart from the functional diagrams and CT's outstanding utility in renal studies (which are performed as serial studies, usually with contrast media), morphological studies are also carried out which can reveal perirenal hematomas, abscesses, kidney urinary stasis, uroceles, lymphoceles and cysts. Serial studies, which can be performed for the whole body [15] (brain, coronary artery bypass, pulmonary, hepatic, pancreatic and even eye studies), involve the use of a relatively high radiation dose, so these studies should be planned properly.

21.5 Pelvic studies

The organs and bones in the pelvic cavity can be studied using CT. The diseases of the bladder, large intestine and testis, and retroperitoneal tumors, tumors of the lymphatic system (lymphoma), etc, are among the conditions that can be evaluated with this technique.

Figure 21.17 shows an intra-abdominal lymphoma that affects internal organs with various lesions marked with arrows.

It should be clarified that studies of the lymphatic system can result in misdiagnosis [16], due to a set of anatomical and technical factors beyond the scope of this book. Therefore, knowledge of the literature and the experience accumulated by experts are necessary to recommend the procedures and techniques necessary to achieve the expected results.

References

[1] Ambrose J and Gooding M 1976 EMI scan in the management of head injuries *Lancet* **307** 847

[2] Lanksch W, Oettinger W and Bethmann A 1977 Diagnosis of brain edema using CT *J. Comput. Assisted Tomogr.* **1** 13–19

[3] Heller M, Jend H, Grabbe E and Hambuchen K 1981 Tomografía computarizada seriada *Electromédica* **2** 68–72

[4] Bartlett J and Neil-Dwyer G 1978 A clinical study of the EMI scanner implications of neuroradiological services *Br. Med. J.* **2** 813

[5] Luft Ch Trenkler J 1986 Localización de procesos craneales por tomografía axial computarizada *Electromédica* **3** 166–9

[6] Kuhler W 1978 CT scanning of the thorax *Xtract*

[7] Kang M J and Park C M *et al* 2010 Dual-energy CT: clinical applications in various pulmonary diseases *Radiographics* **30** 685

[8] Lipson S 2005 *Clinical Advancements in Volumetric CT, Data Overload* (Tokyo: Toshiba Medical Systems)

[9] Cronqvist S, Bmsmar J, Kjeillin K and Soderstrom C 1975 Computer assisted axial tomography in brain-vascular lesions *Acta Radiol. Scand.* **16** 135–42

[10] Rogalsky W and Hahn R 1982 Técnica cardiográfica con el somatom *Electromédica* **2** 51–61

[11] Inamoto K, Kawakita S and Shimizu Y 1982 Reconstrucción de transplantes de bypass aortocoronarios en tomogramas computarizados *Electromédica* **1** 11–19

[12] Fuchs H 1976 Whole body computer tomography selected findings from the abdominal area *Electromédica*

[13] Hammerschlag S, Wolpert S and Carter B 1987 Computed tomography of the spinal canal *Radiology* **121** 361–9

[14] Jeschke G and Will H 1985 Tomografía computarizada seriada cuantitativa *Electromédica*

[15] Vankaick G, Jaschke W and Strauss I 1979 The relationship between ultrasonography and computed tomography in the diagnostic examination *Electromédica* **3** 109–17

[16] Kreel L 1976 The EMI whole body scanner in the demonstration of lymph node enlargement *Clin. Radiol.* **27** 421–9

IOP Publishing

Technical Fundamentals of Radiology and CT

Guillermo Avendaño Cervantes

Chapter 22

Other specialized studies

22.1 Introduction

Previous chapters have described the basic functions and main applications of CT, however there are further, less common, applications [1], which have great potential for future development, such as the following:

- Pulmonary studies [2].
- Pelvimetry using topograms.
- Three-dimensional bone reconstruction.
- Three-dimensional vascular reconstruction.
- Mineral densitometry.
- Abdominal trauma.
- Precision cineradiography.
- Cerebral dynamics using xenon.
- Stent installation.

Because these are not very common procedures, we will only give a basic description and show images of some of these specialized studies.

22.2 Pelvimetry using topograms

Designed in 1982, pelvimetry using topograms consists of using images based on topograms of the pelvic region in pregnant women who require an exact determination of the cephalo–pelvic relationship. That is, this technique can determine if the proportions of the fetal head in relation to the opening of the bones of the pelvis require a cesarean section or if vaginal delivery is possible. This method [3] surpasses conventional pelvimetry in accuracy and is performed over a shorter time, and has the specific important advantage that the collimation procedure allows lower irradiation of the patient and the fetus.

The images and measurements made by the computer can both be obtained axially with a tomogram in the form of digital radiography (a topogram).

doi:10.1088/978-0-7503-1212-7ch22

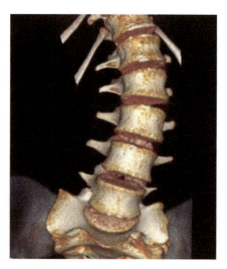

Figure 22.1. A three-dimensional image of vertebrae. Courtesy of Siemens.

22.3 Three-dimensional reconstruction

Obtaining an image showing a three-dimensional organ, bone, or any structure under study is an extraordinary aid in the diagnosis process. The software created for this function uses axial scans, reconstructing volume bodies with any inclination and perspective. This delicate and advanced application, which was initially regarded with great hopes of promising results [4], is now fortunately an important reality.

The case of spinal reconstruction is remarkable. Back pain caused by herniated nuclei, spinal fusion processes in vertebrae, spinal stenosis, herniated discs, etc, are the most spectacular of these studies [5] and the results are obvious, even to non-specialists (see figure 22.1). The unification of the axial images in a volume [6], allows one to see the object under study in a similar way as observed in surgical exploration, with the important advantage of eliminating or adding to neighboring or intermediary structures. Thus parts of the spine can be represented showing vertebrae and their relationships.

The three-dimensional analysis of head tomograms (the bones of the face) is also used to good effect in accurately planning surgery [7], as shown in figure 22.2.

22.4 Densitometry of bone mineral content

This application of densitometry uses at least two energy levels of x-rays to assess the content of different minerals [8] in the bones to be examined. An immediate application of this technique is the study of osteoporosis, a widespread metabolic disease among the elderly, which is characterized by the reabsorption of the calcified bone matrix occurring faster than the tissue reconstruction. Osteoporosis leads to reduced bone mass and high fracture incidence. Although the treatment of this disease remains controversial, the proper diagnosis is currently made using quantitative densitometry with CT [9].

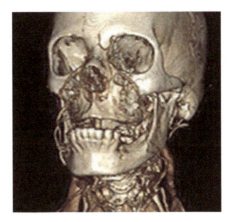

Figure 22.2. Three-dimensional reconstruction of facial bones. Courtesy of Siemens.

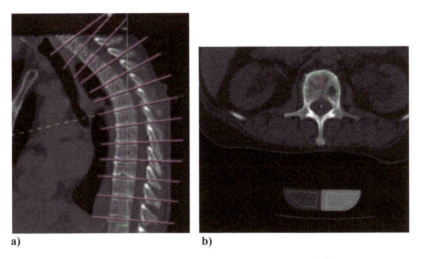

Figure 22.3. Bone mineral quantitative CT. Courtesy of Siemens.

Figure 22.3(a) shows a topographical sagittal image with indicators of different levels of mineral content [10], reflected in the numerical levels, while in the axial image on the right (b) reference the mineral content of the vertebras displayed in the phantom outlined below the patient.

22.5 Studying abdominal trauma using CT

The viscera and internal organs of the abdominal cavity may be injured in diverse ways when severe trauma occurs [11]. Before the application of CT, diagnostic techniques were complex and depended on a set of procedures such as excretory urography, angiography, laparoscopic studies (an exploratory form of endoscopy) and enteroclysis. All of these procedures involve delays that risk the patient's condition worsening, in addition to being generally painful or bothersome to the patient [12].

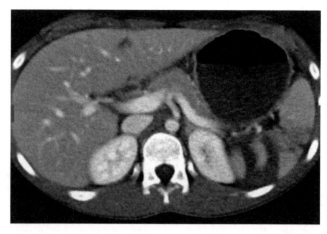

Figure 22.4. Images of abdominal trauma using CT. Courtesy of Siemens.

Because abdominal injuries are usually the result of accidents, time is a crucial factor in order to reduce blood loss and progressive deterioration of the patient's general condition. CT allows safe and accurate diagnosis using rapid means, and avoids the need for the repetition of diagnostic measurements, such as angiography, x-rays, etc.

Figure 22.4 shows a case of damage in the pancreas (splenic laceration) by abdominal trauma.

22.6 Cerebral dynamics using xenon

This special form of study involved CT imaging while the patient breathes a mixture of xenon and oxygen [13], which helps in visualizing the physiological processes of blood flow in the brain. This procedure is useful in the case of brain disease or brain vascular accidents, in particular as it provides highly reliable non-invasive results.

The principle of this method is based on the fact that the amount of fluid in a body is determined by the relationship between the fluid given by the arteries and that evacuated through the veins (the Fick principle). Obviously, in diseased tissue, vessels with problems of various kinds (aneurysms, thrombi, etc) produce an appreciable difference compared to the behavior of healthy tissues [14].

Figure 22.5 shows a diagram of the use of a xenon respirator [15] in the top panel, and the bottom panel shows the results of a study, with the anatomical distribution of xenon shown in the brain with a corresponding table of CT numbers and the flow in the region. The left-hand panel of figure 22.6 shows a tomogram of the brain and the right-hand panel the image obtained later.

22.7 CT applications in therapy

CT allows the safe, quick and repeatable calculation of radiation therapy (e.g. cobalt therapy or therapy using accelerated electrons). The CT scan allows an accurate determination of the patient's internal anatomy, and an image and determination of

Technical Fundamentals of Radiology and CT

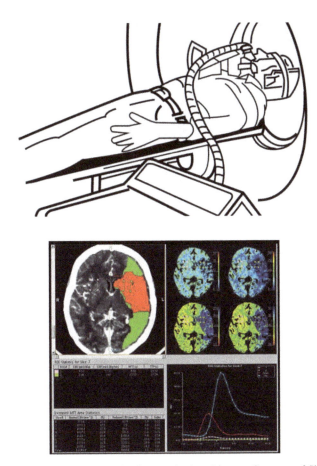

Figure 22.5. A respiratory study diagram (top) and image. Courtesy of Siemens.

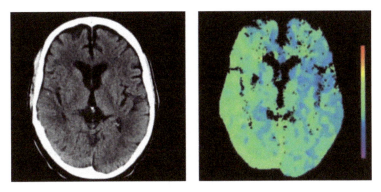

Figure 22.6. Xenon perfusion imaging. Courtesy of Siemens.

the tumor profile. Simultaneously, the physical densities within the stratum can be evaluated to correctly computerized calculations of isodose.

The therapy planning system consists of hardware and software which generally constitute an additional function in CT systems. The software of a therapy planning

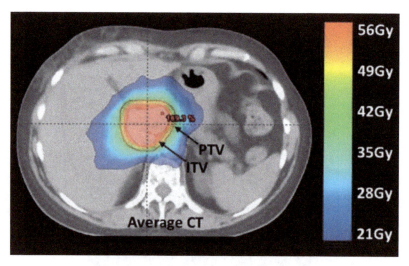

Figure 22.7. Planning radiation therapy. Courtesy of Siemens.

system allows planning for many different types of tumors [16] with different organs programs. These programs may contain:
- External beams of rays.
- Irregular fields.
- Interstitial and intracavitary dosimetry.
- Electron beams.
- Aggregation programs.

Figure 22.7 shows an image obtained with CT in which are superimposed different values of radiation dose to be applied for the treatment of a cancer in the abdominal region.

The therapy planning team uses the high quality images generated by the CT scanner to delineate the tumor and surrounding sensitive tissues [17]. This image superimposes on the tomographic image of the patient a set of values corresponding to isodose, geometric data and distance calculations. These are all available from special software, so that the composite image allows the operator to quickly create a treatment plan for a dose individually compensated at the pixel level. The image can be taken to the screen by means of discs, tapes with multiple images, or through a special frame with the characteristics of a film viewer, on which lines and boundaries are drawn with a special electronic pen that only the operator or the medical physicist uses. Concordance between the radiation beams applied to the patient and their real anatomy is high. This allows the patient to be treated with radiation which will only be applied over the tumor. Figure 22.8 shows a complete therapy planning system [18].

22.8 Installation of stents

Stents are mechanical tubular devices manufactured from specific elastic materials, used to restore the functionality of damaged, tight or collapsed vessels (see figure 22.9).

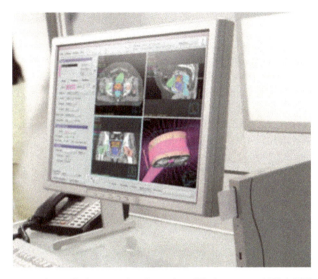

Figure 22.8. A center for radiotherapy planning using CT. Courtesy of Kininklijke Philips N. V.

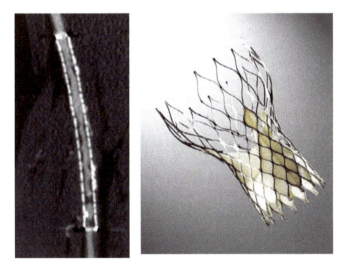

Figure 22.9. Installation of a stent guided by CT (left) and an example of a stent (right). Courtesy of GE.

The morphology of stents allows them to reinforce the structure of the damaged vessel and replace surgical procedures such as bypass installations. For installation, it is necessary for the stent to follow the path of several vessels in collapsed mode and widen in order to acquire the final form when it arrives at the installation site [19], strengthening the affected vessel. This is achieved using controlling radiation and CT is one of the preferred techniques, the best method is the use of a low radiation dose mode.

References

[1] Alexander J and Krumme J 1988 Somatom plus: nuevas perspectivas en la tomografía computarizada *Electromédica* **2** 50–9

[2] Planz K and Rudiger K 1988 Evaluación de los tomógramas computarizados en presencia de alteraciones fibróticas pulmonares con ayuda de histogramas *Electromédica*

[3] Goldberg H and Federle M 1986 CT pelvimetry *CT Clin. Symp.* **7** 7–9

[4] Roberston D, Fishman E and Walker P 1988 Ambicioso método de formación de imágenes en tomografía computarizada, aplicaciones en la cirugía ortopédica de la cadera *Electromédica* **1** 4–6

[5] Laster R, Bell L and Mills L 1979 Three dimensional CT as an aid in diagnosis of lumbar spine disease after fusion *CT Clin. Symp.* **3** 21–8

[6] General Electric Medical Systems 1987 CT 9000 3-D imaging option *Product Data* **B9800**

[7] Tanaka T, Toyoluku F and Kanda S 1988 Representación tridimensional por TC de las regiones maxilar y facial *Electromédica* **2** 30–9

[8] Saxon R and Bassett L 2002 Osteoporosis: conceptos actuales *Hospimédica* **1** 4–9

[9] Nagel W, Schmidt M, Alexander J and Drexler J 1987 Diagnóstico de la osteoporosis por tomografía computarizada cuantitativa, primeros resultados clínicos *Electromédica*

[10] Reich N and Siedelman F 1976 Determination of bone mineral content using CT scanning *Am. J. Roentgenol.* **127** 593

[11] Federle M 1985 CT of blunt abdominal trauma *CT Clin. Symp.* **9** 17–8

[12] Csendes P, Sanhueza A and Aldana H 2010 Aplicaciones de la tomografía computada multidetector en el estudio del intestino delgado *Rev. Hosp. Clín. Univ. Chile* **17** 279–85

[13] Kashiwagi Sh, Yamashita T, Abiko S, Aoki H and Maekawa L 1986 Medida y visualización del flujo sanguíneo utilizando xenón estable en la tomografía computarizada *Electromédica* **4** 135–9

[14] Lasker R and Bell L 1987 Clinical utility of xenon-CT in cerebral infarction *CT Clin. Symp.* **1** 2–7

[15] Cianfoni A and Colosimo C 2007 Brain perfusion CT: principles, technique and clinical applications *Radiol. Med.* **112** 1225–43

[16] Husband J, Parker R, Cassell C and Hodday P 1978 Radiation therapy planning using a CT 5005 whole body scanner *Xtract* **1** 4–10

[17] General Electric Medical Systems 1986 CT/l' radiotherapy treatment planning *Product Data* **B7900**

[18] EMI Medical 1978 EMI plan 7000 el sistema de planificación de terapia a partir de imágenes TAC *Catalogue* **7000**

[19] Pugliese F and Cademartiri F 2006 Multidetector CT for visualization of coronary stents *Radiographics* **26** 887–904

IOP Publishing

Technical Fundamentals of Radiology and CT

Guillermo Avendaño Cervantes

Chapter 23

Complete tomographic installations

23.1 Introduction

The different components studied in previous chapters make up the complete installations of CT systems, as shown in figure 23.1. The space the installation will occupy needs to be assessed in order to determine the best possible location [1], in addition to which aspects such as electricity, air conditioning, ease of access and removal of patients, etc, need to be considered. All the necessary details can be obtained from the technical information supplied by the manufacturer. Classical installations can be modified in accordance with user requests, always with the intention of allowing fluency in patient care, and the ergonomic installation of components such as the diagnostic console, multi-camera, magnetic memory, film viewer, etc. In considering the design of a facility, it is important to never lose sight of the patient on the diagnosis table, and ensure the possibility of quickly removing the patient in emergency situations and the ability to abort the process when necessary [2]. Devices that are used to perform studies on many patients per day, such as public service institutions or clinics with a very high demand, require superior components, in particular relating to computer memory capacity, so their space requirements are higher than for devices with lower study rates [3].

Currently, the use of high integration electronics enables the manufacture of devices with computer reconstruction and image processing installed in the same operator console, so that the total installed device can comfortably occupy a surface area not exceeding 20 m^2. This means that there is a generation of devices aimed at medium-sized and small clinics that are unable to purchase larger devices, which have almost the same capabilities for handling images and software applications [4]. Figure 23.2 shows a typical installation of a small system [5]. It can be seen that, in the same room where the patient table (2) and gantry (1) are located, one can find the radiological generator (4) and the high voltage transformer (3), hidden by a decorative panel. The operator console (5) with the computer is housed in a separate

doi:10.1088/978-0-7503-1212-7ch23

© IOP Publishing Ltd 2016

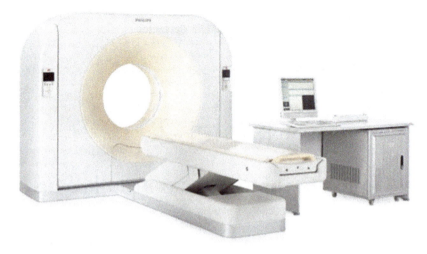

Figure 23.1. A large CT device installation. Courtesy of Koninklijke Philips N.V.

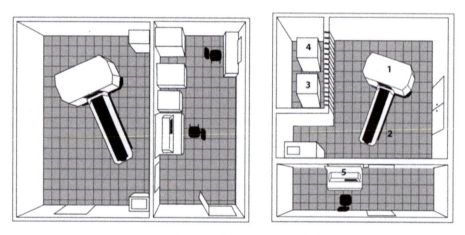

Figure 23.2. A small CT system installation.

room, along with a wall film viewer, a printer and some furniture for different purposes, completing this simple, but modern, facility.

23.2 Mobile CT devices

Sometimes the requirements for CT systems cannot be met by all small hospitals or clinics, despite the existence of compact systems with lower cost and lower installation requirements (space, civil engineering, energy, etc). One of the solutions found in many countries is to share a mobile device between several medical centers [6] providing services to different institutions according to an agreed program. This is essentially a mobile CT device on wheels that travels between clinics, which can sometimes be considerably larger than the usual compact systems.

This method has other advantages. First, the device travels to the patient, thereby reducing transportation costs for ambulances and personnel. Moreover, the devices can be used to conduct studies or research on specific population groups or inhabitants of a given region. These systems, which are manufactured by specialized firms [7], can be of two forms: in-vehicle devices, such as that shown in figure 23.3, or devices installed in an enclosure that is towable by almost any suitable carrier (figure 23.4). Both these types of units are equipped with heating and air conditioning and can quickly and easily connect to previously prepared electrical connections. Current technological developments are focused on achieving faster processes, in order to obtain as many

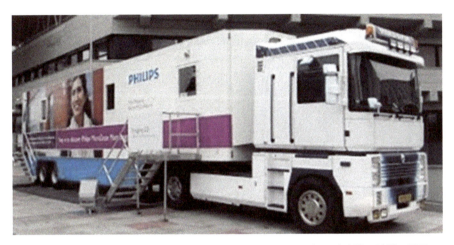

Figure 23.3. External views of a mobile CT device. Courtesy of Koninklijke Philips N.V.

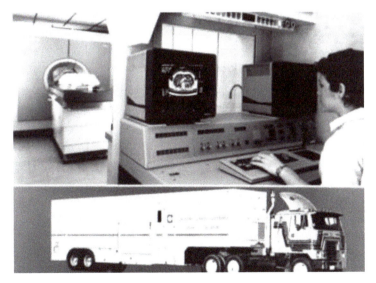

Figure 23.4. Internal and external views of a mobile CT device. Courtesy of Philips.

images as possible, and optimizing the quality of the results, while reducing the cost of devices and radiation doses. Thus, any innovation is beneficial for patients.

References

[1] General Electric Medical Systems 1986 T 9000 series I scanner systems *Product Data* B7960AE

[2] General Electric Medical Systems 1987 The new CT 9000 series from General Electric *Catalog* 5867

[3] General Electric Medical Systems 1989 CT/T scanner system *Product Data* B7800A

[4] General Electric Medical Systems 1987 Mobile CT a cost effective approach to high quality health care *Report*

[5] General Electric Medical Systems 1987 CT Max scanner system *Product Data* B7940HA

[6] Calumet Coach Company 1990 The complete mobile shared CT system *Report*

[7] Toutenkamion Product Data http://www.toutenkamion.com/specific-medical-units.html

IOP Publishing

Technical Fundamentals of Radiology and CT

Guillermo Avendaño Cervantes

Chapter 24

Digital radiography

24.1 The development visualization with x-rays

The image intensifier was developed in the 1950s. This was a breakthrough because it inaugurated the process of fluoroscopy with CCTV, as discussed in chapter 10. Previously a fluorescent screen was used, which has today been eliminated due to its low image quality and, in particular, the risk to the observer who was in the path of the x-rays, despite leaded glass being used to observe the screen. With the image intensifier, it was possible to achieve a marked increase in image brightness and improved security for the physician or technologist operating the device.

For decades, improvements to systems fell within the same concepts, using image intensifiers and TV circuits. However, the appearance of CT and the related digital processes allowed the elimination of radiographic film and all related items [1], such as the cassette, the developer, developer chemicals, the dark room and the film viewer box. Images could now be produced and viewed directly on computer screens, printed on paper to obtain hard copies and be sent to remote locations using digital media, such as the Internet or satellite systems.

In the 1980s digital subtraction angiography (DSA) was developed, which is preferably applied in cardiovascular examinations and in contrasted encephalic vessels. In DSA, the analog video signals obtained from an image intensifier and a special TV camera become two scanned images with and without contrast, which can be compared in a point-by-point mode by a computer, allowing the exclusive observation of vessels filled with contrast medium. This allows the very accurate diagnosis of vascular conditions as the exclusive image of narrowing vessels, occlusions, aneurysms, stroke or any other pathological condition is so clearly identified and defined in space.

New advances were sought in technological methods which would obtain digital images regardless of the film and could also be achieved without systems that include image intensifiers or all the TV components for fluoroscopy. The solution to these requirements was developed in the 1990s and the early decades of the current

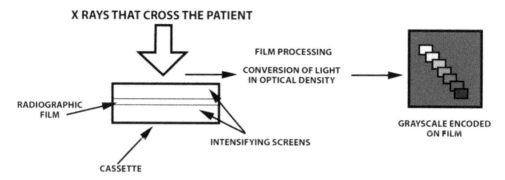

Figure 24.1. A conventional system for obtaining a radiographic image.

century, the great challenge of digital radiography (DR) [2] is currently emerging as methodology used in all medical facilities.

Regardless of current advances, conventional radiography remains an option used in contemporary diagnostic procedures, despite the high demand for medical imaging techniques such as CT, MRI, ultrasound, DSA and others. Currently, taking x-rays remains the most used form of diagnostic imaging, even with the appearance of the new technologies; conventional film radiography makes up between 65–70% of all diagnostic imaging studies. Therefore, it is not possible to argue that these other imaging technologies will replace or eliminate the use of conventional radiography. Instead demand has grown in line with the general demands on health services, i.e. it became clear that conventional radiography would continue and this required improvements to increase efficiency. In this context, the possibility of improving the image post-processing, as initiated by CT, became relevant, as did new ways of more efficient archiving, and eventually sending the image using the most current and advanced communication methods, such as satellite tele-transmission and the internet.

The progress of radiography to DR occurred in a natural and progressive way. Computed radiography (CR) became the most popular and economical form, and shaped the transitional step between conventional film radiography and the most advanced DR. Figure 24.1 shows a conceptual diagram of conventional radiography, in which an image is obtained with a gradation of gray tones corresponding to the level of attenuation that the patient interposed between the x-rays and the film has caused.

24.2 Image scan forms

One method of achieving digital images, which is not very widely used, is to obtain x-rays on conventional film which are then scanned by a similar device to those used in most offices to scan images on paper. This can then be shown in a digital format on the computer connected to the scanner. This system does not eliminate the film or the required processing elements, however, it has the advantage that the end of the process produces an image which can be manipulated and transmitted using current digital communication systems [3], which allow the image to be sent to any part of the world for study by specialists. This scanning system is adequate for low-resource and geographically isolated institutions, and obviously does not require radiologists to be on location to interpret the images obtained.

The first attempts to digitize dynamic images [4] were made on the basis of the analog video signal obtained before entering a monitor or from the TV camera screen. As in the scanning systems designed in the 1980s, this device captured the image then made it digital through analog–digital converters, so that the computer processing the image had access to all the possibilities offered by the respective algorithms: displaying window ranges of grayscale images, zooming, digital magnification, freezing the post-processing image, filtering, and all division options and management by software of the results.

24.3 Computed radiography

CR mode digitization of radiographic images has the possibility of using almost any conventional x-ray generator, because it is based on the replacement of the conventional cassette container of radiographic film and intensifying screens by a special device with a similar cassette size [5]. In this cassette there is a sheet of photostimulable phosphor material, known as photostimulable storage phosphor (PSP). When x-rays are received, a latent image is formed which is subsequently recovered by means of a special reading technique using a laser light reader.

CR is a technology that, despite its age, is only made by some manufacturers, particularly companies related to the world of photography such as Fuji, Agfa, Kodak, Konica, Lumisys, ICRco and others. In total there are no more than a dozen providers of this technology.

The plate receiving the radiation is composed of a mixture of barium fluorohalides activated by doped europium. When radiation is applied to one of these plates, the x-rays interact with the phosphor which releases electrons from the impurity atoms. This causes the passage of electrons from the energy levels of the valence band to the energy levels of the conduction band. Many of these electrons are trapped by energy states slightly below the minimum energy of the conduction band and they are retained with a half-life of days. To release these electrons before they spontaneously decay over time, a photon beam with adequate energy must be applied to the phosphor for the electrons to return to the conduction band and be free at the structure. Once free in the conduction band the electrons can decay to the valence band emitting visible light, this occurs when free electrons in the conduction band are captured by impurity atoms of europium that had previously released an electron as a result of the x-ray action, as explained by solid-state theory and shown in figure 24.2.

The light emitted by the plate is converted into an electrical signal by a photomultiplier system, which captures the low light signal and multiplies it, repeatedly generating electric charges that become a current value sufficient to be handled by an amplifier [6]. The set of plate currents realizes the image recorded on the entire surface of the phosphor plate. The red spectral band in the beam of light reaching the photomultiplier tube is removed by a filter to eliminate the light signal

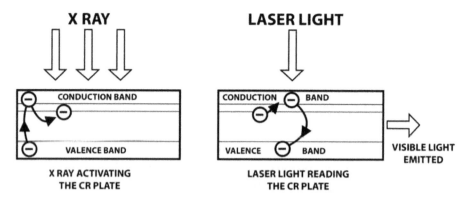

Figure 24.2. The effect on electrons of the x-rays and laser.

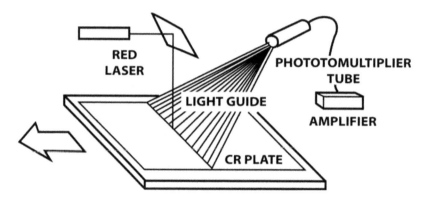

Figure 24.3. A diagram of the reading of scanning plate CR.

from the laser, thus avoiding the background noise that will be captured by the phosphor plate. Figure 24.3 shows a conceptual diagram of the scanning laser beam traversing the plate and 'reading' the latent information.

The image quality [7], in particular the resolution, has to do with the finesse of the laser beam making the scan (see figure 24.4). The more points there are in the matrix, the better the image that is obtained.

The resolution of a radiographic image is critical [8] as the higher the resolution is, the more diagnostic value the image has. Therefore, it is important to ensure that systems have adequate values of line pairs per millimeter (lp mm^{-1}), which are indicated for each type of PSP plate. The instrument used for this measurement is a pattern of line pairs that is exposed to x-rays in conventional imaging, fluoroscopy or DR (see figure 24.5). The resolution level achieved is indicated by the merger of the lines in the obtained image; if the resolution is higher more lp mm^{-1} will be visible.

24.3.1 Advantages of CR

A significant advantage of CR is related to cost reduction, because the PSP plates used in place of conventional film can be used many times without the use of the

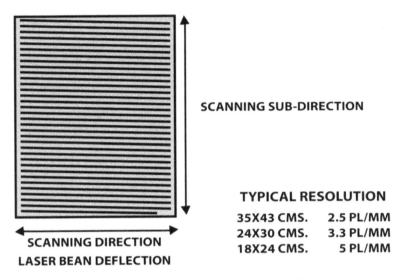

Figure 24.4. Reading with a laser beam and resolutions.

Figure 24.5. An instrument for measuring the lp mm^{-1} of an image.

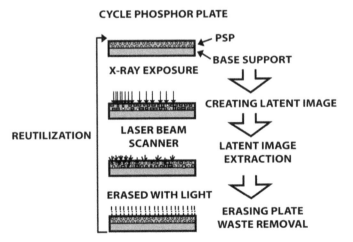

Figure 24.6. The cycle of formation and erasing of an image on the plate.

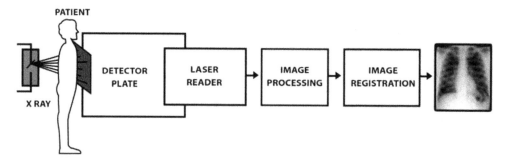

Figure 24.7. A diagram of the general CR system.

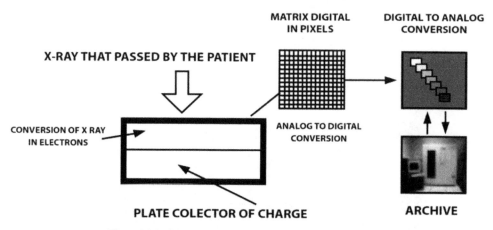

Figure 24.8. A conceptual scheme for obtaining CR images.

consumables required by film, i.e. the developer liquid, developer maintenance, the darkroom and other components. A PSP plate can be used between 15 000 to 40 000 times. Plates are available in different formats in a similar way to cassettes in conventional radiographs. Figure 24.6 shows the formation and erasing of an image on the plate.

Another advantage is the improvement of the efficiency of post-processing. As CR produces a digital image, all kinds of changes can be made, such as improved contrast, digital filtering, magnification, zoom, annotated data, delimiting areas and other modifications, which are applied in several specialties, including dental radiography [9]. The resulting image can be digitally archived, transmitted via an internal network or a global network, and incorporated in online display systems such as radiology information systems (RIS), with all the advantages of sharing different diagnostic images in a protocolized manner.

A distinct advantage of the digital information in images is the fact that the dynamic range of the PSP can achieve more information in an image so that the diagnosis can be made without requiring further radiographic exposures. This brings the additional benefit of the reduction of the radiogenic burden on the patient. In addition, the increasingly improved technology of PSP imaging plates allows a consistent high quality, and improves resolution, the chances of further processing and the speed at which the processes are performed. Diagrams of the general CR system and the conversion process from x-rays in electrical charges, which finally become digital images, are shown in figures 24.7 and 24.8.

24.3.2 Disadvantages of CR

The main disadvantage of CR systems is the need to carry the plate with latent information to the reader and wait for the laser to complete its work in order to obtain the full picture, evaluate its usefulness and perform the possible modifications the digital system allows. Although, this time is shorter than that involved in developing a conventional x-ray film, the speed of CR is limited in comparison to DR.

Another notable drawback is that the system cannot be used to display real-time images such as those obtained in R/F devices where the use of fluoroscopy allows dynamic tracking of a process and the mobilization of dye or the movement of organs like the heart. In other words, CR cannot achieve the equivalent of fluoroscopy.

A factor hindering the introduction and widespread use of CR is resistance to change, a factor that now has less and less influence, because the natural conservatism of people who for many years worked with a technology to which they are accustomed has been modified by the observation of the results. If clinicians, at the beginning of this form of digitization, could object to certain aspects of the digital image not being exactly equal to those obtained by conventional means, the quality of the results now makes it difficult for even the most experienced eye to successfully differentiate between images obtained with conventional techniques and digitized film images printed from multi-format cameras.

Another factor hindering the widespread introduction of CR to replace conventional radiography is the need for operators or users to have some knowledge of computers, or at least the most appropriate use of relevant computer programs for people that do not have access to PC based systems. It can be stressful to learn how to use these kinds of equipment and programs if someone does not feel sufficiently competent.

Many institutions do not incorporate CR or DR systems, as their managers have the perception that the cost is unattainably high. This is because they have not calculated the time to recovery of the money invested, or projected the savings on consumables [10]. Neither have they incorporated into their decision-making the impact of the clinical benefits of having highly manageable images that can be transmitted by various means, the reduction of necessary archive space, development of x-ray film in the machine and, in particular, the increase in the rate of processing of patients due to significant increases in the speed that is achieved in obtaining radiographs and the almost immediate results.

Another limiting factor is often not explicit, but is considered as a possible risk, namely legal information management and the security of what is exchanged between the different specialists and professionals who are, in various ways, involved in obtaining, file handling, transmission and archiving of images. The mere fact that images with the names of patients can be exchanged between computers generates doubts regarding both confidentiality and computer security, although in practical terms security and confidentiality are of a high standard in modern technological systems.

24.4 Digital radiography

Current systems of DR are based on a special panel of fixed dimensions that is mechanically linked in solidarity with the x-ray tube. This creates a substantial difference to CR systems, because the user must purchase the complete system. The generator, including the tube, the collimator and the panel need to be placed in a suitable position to achieve the best conditions for image creation, i.e. suitable magnification, spatial resolution, focus and use of the emission properties of the filament tube.

The alternative to the screens of CR systems [11] are panels which, in principle, should not move anywhere, i.e. fixed panels that can create a digital image through a combination of x-ray conversion into light and solid-state electronics that finally obtain the output digital electrical signals. Thus DR is based on a panel which receives the x-rays and then generates a conversion from light into electrons, which are then manipulated by devices such as high density integrated diodes or transistors.

Such a conversion can be accomplished using two methods, called indirect DR and direct DR. Both systems achieve the conversion of the photons of the x-rays that have impacted on the detection area of each face of the sensor element, constituting the pixel, into an electrical charge stored in the transistor of an active matrix corresponding to each pixel. It is therefore necessary to explain the differences between these two types of digital imaging processes.

24.4.1 Indirect DR

Indirect DR is based on the conversion of x-ray photons into photons of visible light and the subsequent conversion of these photons into electrical charges. The conversion sequence in the indirect method is the following. X-rays impact on a photo-converter plate, i.e. the x-rays impinge on a plate coated with a scintillator substance such as cesium iodide, whereby light is released depending on the intensity of the x-rays. The light is then detected by photodiodes that generate an electrical signal and transfer this to a multitude of tiny transistors called thin film transistors (TFTs), with dimensions of the order of 150 μm × 150 μm, with which a matrix [12] is formed across a panel of fixed dimensions. In the process of x-ray conversion, the light can suffer successive reflections and dispersions in any direction, which means the possibility of losing useful information. This is mathematically accounted for as a reduction in the sensitivity of the system and reduced spatial resolution.

In this last stage the electrical charges that the many transistors handle correspond to the radiation intensity, which is obviously not uniform on the panel surface because the object to be radiographed has different radiation absorption coefficients, as explained in chapter 10. All loads are transferred to a computer that makes an image in the x–y plane as in conventional radiography.

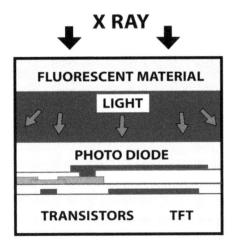

Figure 24.9. A conceptual scheme of indirect DR.

As explained this technology has the drawback of some loss of spatial resolution, but this can be compensated with image re-processing, although with the risk of increasing noise which can also compromise image quality. Figure 24.9 shows the process of creating the image in an indirect DR system.

Based on the above discussion, it is clear that a superior system would be one that could maximize the photoconductivity of conversion for all x-ray photons so as to correspond directly with the generated electrical signals.

24.4.2 Direct DR

The principle of direct DR is based on a fundamental component, generically known as a flat panel, which performs direct conversion [13], i.e. photons of x-rays generate electrical charges that are projected onto an array of TFTs, whereby a signal matrix is generated corresponding to the radiographic image. This is handled by suitable software in order to generate either static or dynamic digital images on a computer. This dynamic methodology has the great advantage that digital images with a better quality spatial resolution than in indirect DR can be obtained.

The main component is the flat panel, an x-ray detector based on direct conversion, with a thickness of 1000 μm using selenium technology (amorphous selenium), enabling DR and fluoroscopy with adequately high resolution. This new type of panel has an area of about 23×23 cm^2 and is made of a photoelectric material and a detector composed of tiny, highly integrated TFTs, the product of advanced solid-state technology. One feature that should be emphasized is the possibility to take fluoroscopic images at 30 frames per second.

The contemporary technological and scientific effort of various manufacturers and researchers aims to achieve both high contrast and high spatial resolution [13], and increase the speed of capture of successive images. These systems can be used

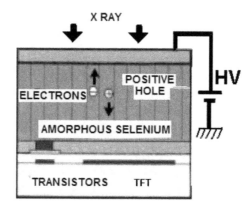

Figure 24.10. A conceptual outline of direct DR.

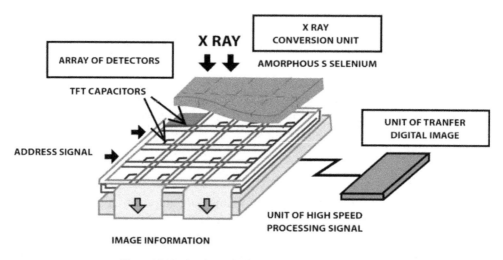

Figure 24.11. A schematic diagram of a classic flat panel.

successfully in general studies, cardiac and cerebral angiography, and conventional gastrointestinal studies. Figure 24.10 shows a conceptual scheme of the conversion of x-rays into electrical signals, and the formation of the image matrix which through software becomes a direct digital image that is shown on the computer screen.

Construction of a flat panel detector
The flat panel [14] consists of four parts: an x-ray conversion unit; a set of tiny solid-state sensors with a high degree of integration; a high-speed processing unit; and a unit for transferring the digital image to the computer. The structure is shown in figures 24.10 and 24.11.

Technical Fundamentals of Radiology and CT

The internal structure and functionality of the flat panel
A photoelectric material is used for x-ray conversion in this unit. Basically, amorphous selenium converts the x-rays that reach the system into small electrical signals. The x-rays arrive at plate coated with a layer of amorphous selenium, where positive and negative charges are created due to the photoelectric properties in a magnitude proportional to the level of radiation. The panel is under a certain level of voltage of the order of several kV, so the electric charges thus generated are moved through the electric field as a photoelectric current and are captured by the detector array.

The detector array
The detectors consist of thousands of transistors constructed with TFT technology, so that a flat panel has more than two million detectors on a crystal substrate. As additional elements with an essential role in the operation of the detector, a capacitor and tiny TFTs are included. When x-rays impact on the detectors, charges that accumulate in the capacitor are generated. When a TFT is initialized by a signal from the high speed processing unit, the accumulated charges are converted into an electrical signal which, together with the other electrical signals, creates the image.

The high-speed processing unit for signals
This unit carries out the conditioning of the electrical signals coming from the sensors [15] so that they are converted into digital values by the incorporated analog–digital converter. The processing methodology involves sequentially activating the TFTs of the detector array by the arrival of pulses generated in the sequencer. The electrical signals resulting from this activation are amplified and sent to an analog–digital converter as shown figure 24.12.

The main difference between indirect and direct DR [16] is the signal quality which ultimately leaves the panel. In the first case the signal, generated by a system consisting of a cesium iodide scintillator and its manipulation by means of photo-diodes and TFTs, has a profile with a flared shape and is therefore less efficient in

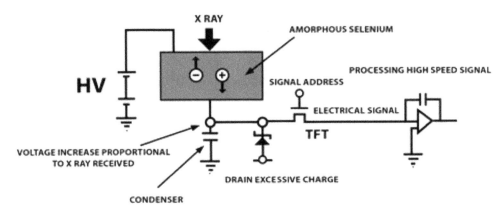

Figure 24.12. An electronic scheme of x-ray conversion into charges and voltages proportional to the radiation.

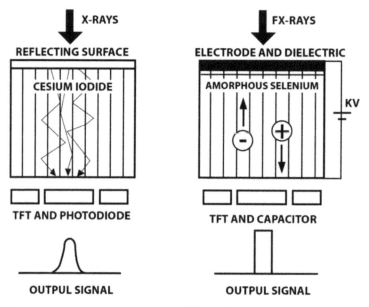

Figure 24.13. A comparison of indirect and direct DR in relation to the quality of the output signal.

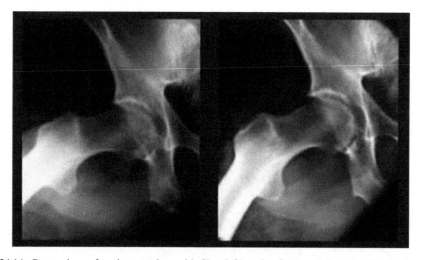

Figure 24.14. Comparison of an image taken with film (left) and a flat panel detector (right). Courtesy of Philips.

terms of spatial resolution. The output signal of the flat panel of amorphous selenium, on the other hand, is more efficient because its profile is rectangular and uniform, as shown in figure 24.13.

Finally, we note that in clinical practice, the results of DR systems are completely adequate for use of the obtained image in accurate diagnosis. Figure 24.14 shows a comparison between a conventional film x-ray image with film and that of a DR system, showing the advantage of the digital image [17].

References

[1] Medical Imaging 2002 Living the digital vision *Product Data*

[2] Schaefer-Prokop C and Prokop M 1997 Digital radiography of the chest: comparison of the selenium detector with other imaging systems *Medicamundi* **41** 2–11

[3] Multi Diagnostic Imaging Systems 2006 OREX ACLXY™ specifications *Product Data*

[4] Hamers S and Freyschmidt J 1998 Digital radiography with an electronic flat-panel detector: first clinical experience in skeletal diagnostics *Medicamundi* **42** 2–6

[5] MacMahon G H 2003 Digital chest radiography: practical issues *J. Thoracic Imaging* **18** 124–37

[6] Eastman Kodak Company 2011 Directview DR 9000 system *Product Data*

[7] Eastman Kodak Company 2003 Introducing the digital future of imaging *Health Imaging Division Course*

[8] Eastman Kodak Company 2011 Direct view Capturelink system *Product Data*

[9] Orex Computed Radiography 2010 Orex computed radiography for dental practices *Product Data*

[10] Foos D H 2004 Power of digital x-ray boosts workflow *Diagn. Imaging* **1** 1–4

[11] Eastman Kodak Company 2009 Site planning for the Kodak Direct-View DR 5100 system *Product Data*

[12] Eastman Kodak Company 2012 Direct-View DR 7500 system *Product Data*

[13] Hamers S and Freyschmidt J 1998 Digital radiography with an electronic flat-panel detector: first clinical experience in skeletal diagnostics *Medicamundi* **42** 2–6

[14] Neitzel U 1997 Integrated digital radiography with a flat electronic detector *Medicamundi* **41** 2–11

[15] Lot Oriel Group 2012 X-ray CCD detector *Course Notes*

[16] Eastman Kodak Company 2010 Introduction to digital, the role of digital radiography in medical imaging *Health Imaging Division Course*

[17] Neitzel U 2001 X-ray today *Medicamundi* **45** 88–113

IOP Publishing

Technical Fundamentals of Radiology and CT

Guillermo Avendaño Cervantes

Chapter 25

Mammography in three dimensions

25.1 Justification for the method

Breast cancer is the most common cause of cancer death among women and the most frequently diagnosed cancer in women in 140 of 184 countries worldwide [1]. Mortality is higher in less developed countries due to a lack of early detection and access to appropriate treatment.

Three-dimensional (3D) tomosynthesis uses a very powerful device to convert digital breast images into a succession of very thin layers [2], which form a 3D image of the breast. During the examination, the articulated arm of the device follows an arched path over the breast, taking multiple images of each breast in only seconds. Then, a sophisticated computer generates a 3D image of the breast tissue that allows the millimeter scale analysis of layers and high-resolution analysis to be carried out at the same time.

Now doctors can analyze breast tissue with a greater level of detail than ever before. Instead of seeing the complex composition of breast tissue in a flat image, he/she can now examine the breast 1 mm at a time. Small details can no longer hide in the surrounding tissue as now everything will be perfectly visible. This method allows the layer-by-layer analysis of breast tissue while avoiding overlapping. This reduces false positives, i.e. diagnoses of cancer that is actually not present, and false negatives, which are more harmful as they indicate the absence of malignancy despite the presence of true cancer tissue [3].

A major advantage of 3D mammography is that having a better diagnosis reduces the number of complementary studies required for patients. Digital breast tomosynthesis (DBT) is seen as a complement and/or alternative to mammography in the diagnosis of breast cancer in both mass screening programs and in the case of women with suspected cancer. 3D tomosynthesis is very similar to digital mammography, and takes about the same time. The patient needs only to attend the study without powder or deodorant on the breast or armpit.

doi:10.1088/978-0-7503-1212-7ch25   25-1   © IOP Publishing Ltd 2016

The study can be carried out in three ways:
- Unilateral: only one breast. Bilateral: both breasts.
- Magnified: to obtain greater detail in questionable areas.
- The Eklund technique: for patients with breast implants, this technique consists of stretching the breast tissue, leaving the prosthesis off the plate of the compression mechanism.

DBT obtained the European Conformity (CE) marking in 2008 for commercial distribution. The technique was reviewed for premarket in the USA in April 2010 by the US Food and Drug Administration (FDA).

It has been found that 3D mammography detects about 30% more hidden cancers [4]. This value increases in screening for breast cancer using DBT, because this technology allows the detection of very early lesions as breast tissue is analyzed millimeter by millimeter, with no overlap. Mammography in 3D can detect smaller cancers at earlier stages, thus reducing the need for the most aggressive treatments for the patients, both in terms of surgical and oncological approaches.

This technique can reduce or eliminate overlap and differentiate tissue structures in different planes. Tomosynthesis provides a new technology based on imaging of the compressed breast from multiple angles by scanning with an x-ray tube, to subsequently reconstruct an image with 1 mm thick slices. The most common radiological pattern showing the presence of tumors is the star pattern. The star pattern and tumors are associated with micro-calcifications which appear in 100% of cases of breast cancer.

25.2 The aims of tomosynthesis

The optimal use of 3D mammography devices is aimed at achieving:
- Images with the best quality possible to locate lesions for treatment or biopsy.
- Application of the lowest possible radiation dose to patients.
- Cancer screening at a subclinical stage (the detection of tumors 10 mm or less in size is connected to a high survival rate).

The average age for patients diagnosed with breast cancer is 52.9 years and the risk of breast cancer increases from the age of 40 onward. 95% of cancer cases are invasive and only 5% are carcinomas *in situ*. Adding tomosynthesis to conventional 2D mammography showed an increase in the detection rate from 1.3% to 2.57% [5]. DBT is a valid diagnostic test that improves the detection of nodules, reduces the effects of overlapping tissue and facilitates morphological analysis thereof, in particular in dense breasts where the risk of cancer is greater.

Mammography is the imaging technique used in the screening of asymptomatic breast tumor pathology. It is useful in the evaluation of malignant lesions, which manifest as spiculated nodules, architectural distortions and asymmetries, but in some breast parenchyma these injuries may go unnoticed due to the high density of glandular tissue, which can mask signs of cancer.

25.3 A comparison of 2D mammography and 3D DBT

2D mammography is a method that allows the image to be captured with the highest resolution and with the least amount of radiation—a dose of about 0.7 mSv. Its ability to identify lesions of minimum size allows its use in systematic detection of tumors before they become palpable and clinically evident (mammography screening). The scientific evidence shows that mammography screening reduces mortality from breast cancer by an average of 24% (18–30%).

The procedure is performed through two projection routines: cranio–caudal projection (CC) and medio–lateral oblique projection (MLO). These complement each other and help to locate lesions spatially, because breasts consist of different fibroglandular structures that have very similar densities. Therefore an optimized technique is needed to create the maximum possible contrast between small density differences. Modern mammography can detect very small lesions about 5 mm in size, which are impossible to palpate, and microcalcifications (under 1 mm) that are a key element in the early detection of breast cancer, as 71% of so-called 'minimum breast cancers' are diagnosed from their presence alone.

One of the most common limitations are radiologically dense breasts, which are composed almost primarily of dense glandular tissue (common in younger women). This is why mammography should not be applied in patients under 35–40 years, in accordance with expert opinion, because malignant lesions can be very difficult to distinguish from the surrounding normal tissue, because it does not offer sufficient contrast to make lesions visible [6].

3D digital mammography or tomosynthesis (DBT) of the breast is a technique for obtaining a 3D image of the breast based on a modification of digital mammography. The system consists of an x-ray tube installed in a rotational system, which rotates along a certain angle which may range from 15–50°. This movement can take 60 to 70 projections in two dimensions (in 10–20 s) to create tomograms (also called cuts or slices) of 1 mm in any plane, allowing anatomical breast reconstruction in 3D. The images obtained can be presented in individual cuts as in digital mammography, as CC or MLO cuts, or images in a video file.

25.4 How to perform mammography

The procedure for DBT is similar to a digital mammography. The breast is compressed in a table containing a full-field detector with the following characteristics:

- High detective quantum efficiency (DQE).
- A direct converter in an amorphous selenium panel.
- An LCD screen with a range of 2816 × 3584 pixels.
- 85 micro-pixels in an area of 23.9 cm × 30.5 cm.
- High speed for low noise digital images.
- Optimized time detector readings.
- 25 projections over an angular range of 50° should be acquired with full resolution within about 20 s in current devices.

25.5 The image acquisition protocol

The protocol for performing tomosynthesis of four projections in bilateral 2D mammography, with its respective 3D mammography (tomosynthesis), is the following:
  - CC in the right breast in 2D and 3D (tomosynthesis).
  - CC in the left breast in 2D and 3D (tomosynthesis).
  - MLO in the right breast in 2D and 3D (tomosynthesis).
  - MLO in the left breast in 2D and 3D (tomosynthesis).

In general, mammographic studies have three stages [7]:
  1. Acquisition of the image. The image display is performed using one to three projections, in the CC, MLO and Eklund techniques. The number of cuts is defined according to the type of study and conditions of the patient. It is necessary to manipulate and compress the breast during the procedure.
  2. Image processing.
  3. Presentation and interpretation of images.

25.6 Compressing the breast

Compression is performed for the following reasons:
  - To standardize the thickness of the breast tissue.
  - To reduce the radiation dose.
  - To prevent movement of the breast.
  - To separate the structures and reduce overlap.

25.7 DBT devices

Due to the special nature of DBT, the devices used have significant similarities to and some differences from the conventional mammography devices described in chapter 4. The system consists of a general support and a computerized workstation. The general support has an attached platform where the x-ray tube with its rotational system is located, the base where the breast of the patient is placed (there are special plates for breast compression) and an image detector (see figure 25.1). The span of the system is 235 cm high and 117.5 cm wide.

The x-ray tubes used in most types of devices have a rotating anode facing at an angle to the cathode where the electrons generating the x-rays are emitted. However, in the tubes used in mammography, the anode has two angled tracks and two filaments per track, making mammographic tubes unique. The electron emitter of the tube is similar in both cases and a very fine filament is required. The anode must also be made up of two different types of track, one of molybdenum and the other of rhodium. Different combinations of anode and filter are also used, i.e. dual anode filters Mo–Mo or Mo–Rh. The filters help reduce the radiation that is useless for image formation.

The main difference is the angular displacement of the tube around the breast of the patient, similar to the concept explained for linear tomography devices. The different sections that make up the tomosynthesis allow the differentiation of

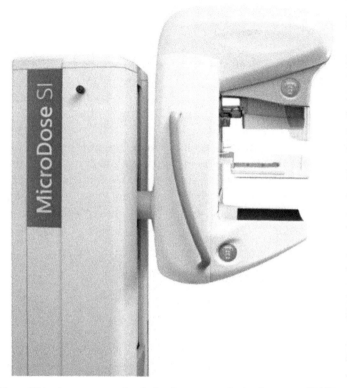

Figure 25.1. A mammography device for tomosynthesis. Courtesy of Philips.

structures in the images to be achieved. This is shown in figure 25.2, where the difference can be seen between two projections at different angles, which will directly affect the depth of resolution. Two projections of ±7.5° may not be able to separate the two spheres shown in the image on the left. Two projections of ±25°, if they can separate the two spheres, allow a depth that gives the proper resolution [8].

25.7.1 Technical specifications

The basic requirements for all mammography systems are [9]:
- High tension (a kVp tube).
- A fine filament (the source of emission).
- An anodic track and filters (radiation quality).
- Appropriate mAs values (current and time values, contrast and optical density).
- A compression mechanism (to achieve radiation uniformity).
- Collimation (delimitation of x-rays on the breast).
- Automatic exposure control (AEC; automatic adjustment of optimal radiation).
- Tomographic movements from 5° to 50°.

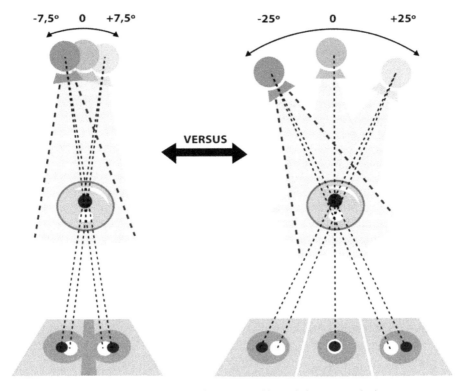

Figure 25.2. The effect of the tomographic angle in tomosynthesis.

25.7.2 Generator requirements

The following are the requirements for the x-ray generator in mammography:
- Output power 5–7 kW.
- kV range 20–40 kV (adjustable in increments of 1 kV).
- Range of mAs to 25 kV and maximum power with a molybdenum anode: 2–500 mAs in mAs mode; 5–500 mAs in AEC mode.
- Range of mAs to 25 kV and maximum power with tungsten anode: 2–630 mAs in mAs mode; 5–630 mAs in AEC mode.
- Exposure time: 10 ms–4 s (large focus); 60 ms–6 s (small focus).

25.7.3 X-ray tube requirements

The following are the requirements for the x-ray tube in mammography:
- A rotating anode tube (tungsten, molybdenum).
- A small focal point value.
- Focal point for molybdenum: 0.1/0.3 (star pattern); 0.15/0.3 (IEC 336).
- Focal point for tungsten: 0.1/0.3 (star pattern); 0.15/0.3 (IEC 336).
- A nominal voltage of 40 kV.
- Heat storage capacity for molybdenum: 1 800 000 J; 2 430 000 HU.
- Heat storage capacity for tungsten: 120 000 J; 162 000 HU.

- An optical anode angle of 20°.
- Inherent filtration of 1 mm Be.
- An anode rotation speed of 8 800 rpm.

25.7.4 Requirements for tomosynthesis

The following are the requirements for DBT:
- Scan angle: ±25°.
- Scan time: <25 s.
- Number of projections: 25.
- Slice acquisition rate: 1.25 projections per second.
- Reconstruction time: ~60 s.
- Distance between reconstructed slices: 1 mm.
- Analytical reconstruction algorithms.
- Data volume projection: 20 MB.

25.7.5 Verification testing of mammographic devices

The following tests should be performed according to a calibration protocol to ensure proper functioning of the system and above all, the quality of the images:
- Physical inspection of devices.
- Focus evaluation of tube (size and resolution, using a star pattern and pinhole).
- Collimation (accuracy).
- Evaluation of voltage (consistency and reproducibility).
- Evaluation of beam quality (thickness half value reduction).
- Evaluation of automation of AEC.

25.8 Qualitative analysis of the image

To optimize the work of a DBT device it is necessary that all technical aspects are properly adjusted to achieve the best quality of mammographic images [10]. The basic factors in image quality are:
- Resolution, depending on the size of the focus.
- Contrast, determined by the quality of the radiation and tissue density.
- Noise, determined by technical factors such as the sensitivity of the digital receptor.

25.8.1 Focus calculation and measuring instruments

The following equation is used to determine the optimal size of the focal spot:

$$f = \frac{\pi\theta}{180} \times \frac{D_{\mathrm{blur}}}{(M_{\mathrm{star}}-1)}$$

where:

D_{blur} = diameter of blurring;

M_{star} = magnification factor, determined by measuring the diameter of the star pattern on the acquired image;

θ = angle of the radiopaque angular sectors (0.5–1°).

Technical Fundamentals of Radiology and CT

The following are the sizes of focal spot accepted by the International Electrotechnical Commission (IEC):
- A focal spot of 0.3 mm cannot generate an image star pattern greater than 0.45 mm wide and 0.65 mm long.
- A focal spot of 0.4 mm cannot generate an image star pattern greater than 0.60 mm wide and 0.85 mm long.
- A focal spot of less than 0.3 mm is an optimal value.

25.8.2 How to use a pinhole camera

In figure 25.3 the following equation is used in conjunction with that obtained with the pin hole camera:

$$\sigma = \frac{\sqrt{12}}{4\pi} \frac{\lambda}{w} d.$$

25.8.3 Quality for diagnostics

A CC image must meet the following quality parameters, as numbered in figure 25.4:
1. A clear display of the pectoral muscle on the side of the image.
2. A clear display of retro-glandular fat.

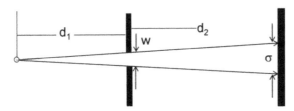

Figure 25.3. Use of a pinhole camera.

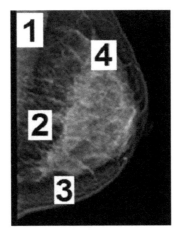

Figure 25.4. Quality parameters in a CC image.

3. A clear display of medial breast tissue.
4. A clear view of the lateral glandular tissue.

25.8.4 Ranges of gray in images

Computed radiography uses 12 bits of depth, which gives the digital image a range of 4096 shades of gray. It is a well-known concept in all digital imaging systems that a greater range of gray values, corresponding to powers of 2, produces better image quality.

25.8.5 The relation between malignancy and information in the image

The Breast Imaging Reporting and Data System (BI-RADS) is a quality assurance tool designed to standardize mammography reporting. It provides a range of seven numbers to describe the level of malignancy of the findings made with mammography. The system consists of several sections, which from a practical point of view can be grouped into descriptions of mammographic lesions (parameters of the masses, calcifications, special cases found and associated findings), and recommendations based on the degree of suspicion for malignancy.

The BI-RADS system defines seven categories of suspects, one of which (category 0) is an incomplete assessment category mainly used for screenings which need more information to determine the appropriate clinical attitude and/or diagnosis; the rest of the categories have full evaluations [11]. The categories describe the possibility of finding different conditions such as distortion of architecture, irregular nodules, calcifications, asymmetries, nodular opacity, high density masses, speculated form (like a star), benign nodes, surrounded node conduits, microcalcifications and others, all of which can be observed on a screen that shows multiple images simultaneously, as seen in figure 25.5.

BI-RADS categories:
- 0: Incomplete.
- 1: Negative.
- 2: Benign findings.
- 3: Probably benign.
- 4: Suspicious abnormality.
- 5: Highly suspicious of malignancy.
- 6: Known biopsy with proven malignancy.

25.9 Safety and radiation doses in DBT

For radiation safety in tomosynthesis it is necessary to understand specific concepts, such as mean glandular dose, a dosimetric quantity generally recommended for risk assessment. This is calculated using phantoms and through specialized algorithms as shown in figure 25.6, in which the position of the phantom and the image obtained by making a radiographic exposure on this simulated breast tissue is shown. For a satisfactory test using a phantom, 80% of the fibers, grains and masses present in the phantom should be detected.

The mean glandular dose is a fundamental measurement to obtain high quality mammography [12]. The performance of AEC relates to the necessary dose (the

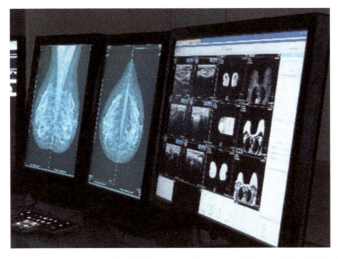

Figure 25.5. A photograph of a DBT station. Courtesy of Koninklijke Philips N.V.

mean glandular dose) in mGy relative to the thickness of the breast tissue. The radiation dose is a major concern for the International Commission on Radiological Protection (ICRP) due to the potential risks of ionizing radiation. For a breast which is about 5 cm thick and has a 50% glandular fraction, the dose in tomosynthesis

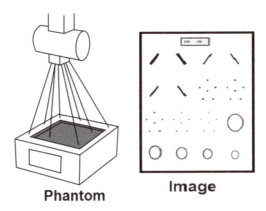

Figure 25.6. The use of a phantom for quality testing in mammography.

imaging is only 8% higher compared to analog mammography and digital mammography (1.3 mGy to 1.2 mGy, respectively). Tomosynthesis is considered a safe procedure [13], because the radiation doses used are within the ranges established by the Mammography Quality Standards Act (MQSA).

Spatial resolution is determined using an instrument that measures a pair of lines, as described in chapter 24. This test is performed to detect problems of spatial resolution in different parts of the detector. The detectable spatial resolution should be 7 lp mm^{-1}. Finally the compression system must be tested using a special scale to measure the effectiveness of compression, as shown in figure 25.7.

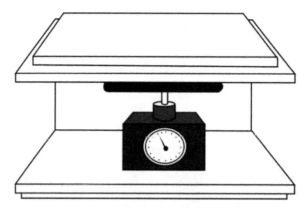

Figure 25.7. The scale for a compression device.

References

[1] World Health Organization 2013 Latest world cancer statistics. Global cancer burden rises to 14.1 million new cases in 2012 *International Agency for Research on Cancer Press Release* 223 https://www.iarc.fr/en/media-centre/pr/2013/pdfs/pr223_E.pdf

[2] Palazuelos G, Trujillo S and Romero J 2014 Breast tomosynthesis: the new age of the mammography *Rev. Colomb. Radiol.* **25** 3926

[3] de Guadalupe Perez M 2014 Valoración diagnóstica de la mamografía 3D (tomosíntesis) en el diagnóstico de cáncer de mama en pacientes mujeres de 40 a 60 años Clínica Internacional—Sede San Borja Año 2013 *Professional Thesis* Universidad Nacional Mayor de San Marcos

[4] Agencia de Evaluación de Tecnologías Sanitarias de Andalucía 2010 Digital tomosynthesis of the breast *Report*

[5] Horvant E, Galleguillos M and Schonteds V 2007 ¿Existen cánceres no detectable en la mamografía? *Rev. Chilena Radiol.* **13** 4429–34

[6] Genaro G *et al* 2010 Digital breast tomosynthesis versus digital mammography: a clinical performance study *Eur. Radiol.* **7** 1545–53

[7] Boyd N F *et al* 2007 Mammographic density and the risk and detection of breast cancer *New Engl. J. Med.* **36** 227–36

[8] Hooley R J *et al* 2012 Screening US in patients with mammographically dense breasts: initial experience with Connecticut Public Act 09-41 *Radiology* **1** 59–69

[9] Baker J A and Lo J Y 2011 Breast tomosynthesis: state-of the-art and review of the literature *Acad. Radiol.* **10** 1298–310

[10] Skaane P *et al* 2013 Comparison of digital mammography alone and digital mammography, plus tomosynthesis in a population-based screening program *Radiology* **1** 47–56

[11] 2000 Guía técnica para el control de calidad de equipos de mamografía *Manual* (Minsal, Cuba)

[12] Karellas A, Vedantham S and Lewin J 2009 Digital mammography: from planar imaging to tomosynthesis *Medicamundi* **53** 14–9

[13] Hakim C M *et al* 2010 Digital breast tomosynthesis in the diagnostic environment: a subjective side-by-side review *Am. J. Roentgenol.* **6** 172–6

CPSIA information can be obtained
at www.ICGtesting.com
Printed in the USA
BVHW011402060222
628173BV00003B/35